LIZ EARLE'S
QUICK GUIDES

Healthy
Menopause

LIZ EARLE'S
QUICK GUIDES

Healthy Menopause

BOXTREE

Advice to the Reader

Before following any dietary advice contained in this book, it is recommended that you consult your doctor if you suffer from any health problems or special condition or are in any doubt.

First published in Great Britain in 1995 by Boxtree Limited, Broadwall House, 21 Broadwall, London SE1 9PL

The right of Liz Earle to be identified as Author of this Work has been asserted by her in accordance with the Copyright, Designs and Patents Act 1988

10 9 8 7 6 5 4 3 2 1

ISBN: 0 7522 1685 6

Text design by Blackjacks
Cover design by Hammond Hammond

Printed and Bound in Great Britain by Cox & Wyman Ltd., Reading, Berkshire

A CIP catalogue entry for this book is available from the British Library

Contents

ACKNOWLEDGEMENTS

I am grateful to Ann Bawtree for helping to produce this book and Leah Wright for her practical help. I am also indebted to the talented team at Boxtree, Rosemary Sandberg and Claire Bowles Publicity, for their unfailing enthusiasm and support.

Introduction

The menopause will affect every woman in her middle years and yet it is not often discussed. Over the last few years the medical world has made great advances in helping many women get through their menopause with greater ease. One of the greatest medical breakthroughs has been the development of HRT, or Hormone Replacement Therapy. Other developments include nutritional knowledge to prevent osteoporosis and surgical operations to treat gynaecological disorders. This *Quick Guide* sets out all the information women need to know about the latest treatments available to them. It also gives an objective view of all the options, clearly listing the pros and cons as they are currently known.

The menopause should not be viewed with dread or fear. With the help of this *Quick Guide*, women will be able to reduce their own menopausal symptoms and be better equipped to cope during this time of natural change.

Liz Earle

—1—

The Menopause, Or 'The Change'

Why the change? There are so many in a woman's life: growing up, education, choice of career, marriage and pregnancy. The menopause is just another of life's milestones and we can all get through it easily with a little care and attention and, if necessary, professional help. It does not have to be dreaded.

Why the dread? In days gone by the onset of menstruation was something to be feared. There were many scare stories of what a girl could expect and how restricted her life would become during 'those days' each month. Now that sanitary protection is advertised nightly on television, the whole world knows that a woman's life does not come to a full stop one week in every four! In fact, in these advertisements menstruating women are portrayed as fitness fanatics who like nothing better than wearing a skin-tight leotard and going roller skating! However, menopausal women do not share this positive image. From some accounts we are led to believe that all women over the age of forty are constantly beset with hot flushes, cold sweats, headaches, indecisiveness, giddy fits, depression, floodings, nervousness, frigidity and middle-aged spread for over a decade until they finally fall into a grey-haired, incontinent heap of disintegrating bones. Look around you. It is just not true!

First of all, the physical facts. Put at its simplest, the menopause marks the end of a woman's fertile years. Her periods stop and she can no longer become pregnant. For many women that is the end of the story, but some will experience unpleasant symptoms, such as insomnia and hot flushes, most of which can be relieved if not completely done away with.

Why does it happen? Well, if it didn't, we would continue to conceive until the grave, and the Family Planning Services would be overstretched to the point of collapse. Unlike the few mature ladies who can afford to go to Italian fertility clinics, Mother Nature realises that babies have the best chance of a normal childhood when born to mothers who can spend the next twenty years of health and energy on their nurture.

The changes of the menopause do not occur suddenly, but develop over a number of years. We all change throughout our lives and many of these changes are brought about by our hormones. These are chemicals made by various glands in our bodies which are released into the bloodstream. The start and finish of a woman's fertile years are governed by hormones. Each month, hormones are made by the pituitary gland in the brain and released into the bloodstream to prompt the ovaries to produce the hormones oestrogen and progesterone. These two hormones have the important job of preparing the lining of the womb to receive a fertilised egg, so that it can grow into a baby. If no egg arrives this lining is shed and is lost in the flow of menstrual blood. After a few days the monthly process restarts. Oestrogen and progesterone are also responsible for puberty. At the menopause this regular monthly cycle finishes.

It might be worth here sorting out exactly what we mean by 'the menopause'. It is a word we are inclined to use rather loosely to mean everything hormonal that happens to a woman in her middle years. The menopause actually means a woman's last period, and she can't know when she has had it until a year or two has passed to prove that it was indeed the last. This is because our periods become very infrequent during the years running up to the menopause. This slowing down process can take as long as five years and has three stages:

Stage one. The first is the 'pre-menopause' and this is the time when the periods first begin both to be less regular in their timing and to vary in heaviness.

Stage two. Then comes the 'peri-menopause', the years when other physical and sometimes psychological alterations are noticed. During the peri-menopause the true menopause occurs and the final period is experienced.

Stage three. The 'post-menopause' refers to the years after the menopause, beginning with the menopause itself and lasting the rest of our days.

The three stages together are known technically as **the climacteric** but in this *Quick Guide* we shall use the term 'menopause'. It is the more usual word, even if it is not what a medical textbook would use.

The only true sign of the menopause is that menstruation stops. This may happen abruptly or, more usually, the periods become more and more irregular, or gradually become lighter and lighter, until they disappear altogether.

If this was all that there is to the menopause, there would be very few women complaining. However, it is reckoned that about 80 percent of women will experience some additional symptoms. Many of these symptoms will be very mild and only very rarely will be so severe that there is little relief. Even in these cases there is the comforting thought that it is, annoyingly, 'only a phase'.

These additional symptoms, discussed in detail in Chapter 2, vary greatly:

* Hot flushes and night sweats (and associated sleep disturbance)
* Incontinence
* Osteoporosis
* Skin and hair problems
* Vaginal dryness and irritation

* Breast problems
* Weight gain
* Depression and changes in mood

But remember – you would have to be one in a million to suffer from *all* of these. You are much more likely to be one of the one in five women who have no noticeable symptoms at all.

The menopause commonly occurs between the ages of forty-five and fifty-five, with the average being fifty-one. It is quite common for it to start in the early forties. Before this, or after the mid-fifties is much less common, but by no means necessarily a cause for concern. The menopause usually lasts for eighteen to twenty-four months.

When the first signs of the menopause begin it is a good idea to make a note of the start date of each period and its duration. This will show how regular or irregular, light or heavy each one is. If a woman is over fifty and has had no period for a whole year, the menopause is considered to be complete. However, in women under fifty, it is wise to allow two years before making any assumptions!

A late, unplanned pregnancy is not everyone's choice. The combined pill is not really suitable for women over the age of forty, or even younger if you are a smoker, because of its associated risk of thrombosis and heart problems. However the mini pill is a good option. There seems to be no evidence that the use of the contraceptive pill affects the onset of the menopause one way or the other. However, it is thought to interfere with the absorption and good effects of nutrients if used over a long time. Coils and IUDs can cause heavy bleeding and so probably the best methods of contraception are the cervical diaphragm or the condom. There is also the possibility of sterilisation.

PREMATURE MENOPAUSE

A very few women experience a natural menopause very early, in their thirties and this tendency runs in families so, if possible, ask your mother about her experiences.

There is substantial evidence that one of the numerous ill-effects of smoking is an unnaturally early menopause.

A more usual cause of premature menopause is due to illness which has necessitated drastic medical treatment. If the ovaries have to be removed or if their function is destroyed, as sometimes happens in cancer treatment, this cuts off the supply of hormones to the womb. The menopause then starts with a bang, bringing on the less desirable effects very suddenly. The removal of the womb does not have such a violent effect if the ovaries can be left in peace to fulfil their purpose.

A twentieth-century phenomenon is the desire to be ultra-thin whilst also being super-fit. Periods can sometimes stop if a woman is undernourished, especially if she is also under great physical stress. If a woman diets excessively and exercises too much, she can become temporarily infertile, which can be reversed with proper nutrition.

Excessive dieting can also cause weakening of the bones, osteoporosis, because the hormones which are responsible for menstruation also keep our bones strong and healthy. This is a very serious matter as bone cannot be replaced once it has been lost.

LATE MENOPAUSE

On the other hand, it is not unknown for some women to have no sign of the menopause until well into their fifties. This too can be quite normal. It is worth having a medical check-up if there is no sign of your periods tailing off by your mid-fifties. If there is 'spotting', (light, scanty periods, especially if accompanied by illness or pain) or any bleeding which occurs at irregular intervals it is important to seek medical help.

Middle Age

The menopause occurs at what we generally call 'middle age', and so the change is going on while much else is happening in our lives. With most people now living much beyond their three score years and ten, middle age must be somewhere between the ages of forty and sixty. What is important is to remember that it is the middle of life, not the beginning of the end. This means that any problems are well worth dealing with because there is a lot of life yet to be lived.

For a mother, this is often the age at which her children are grown and flown, with all the emotional feeling of loss that this can bring. Mothers might console themselves by remembering that charities such as Oxfam and the Cancer Research Campaign would love to achieve what they have. Charities strive to work themselves out of a job by alleviating all the suffering – the reason for their existence in the first place. Similarly, mothers devote eighteen years or more of their lives to creating happy, healthy adults and, once they have reached this goal, their children leave home and put their mothers out of a job. If your children are living independent lives, even if they are not the lives you would have chosen for them, you have done your job well. If you are tempted to think that there is nothing further you can do for them, think again. Even if, at present, they do not need your direct help, you can help them by being happy and fulfilled yourself, so that they do not have to worry about you.

As many women go in for motherhood later in life, the menopause strikes at the time that their offspring are in mid-puberty and enduring the throes of their first hormonal upheaval of life. Well, at least they may be able to sympathise with all the upheaval hormones can cause. For the woman without children, single or married, voluntarily childless or not, the menopause is the time to come to terms with the fact that motherhood is one of the things that is not going to happen to her.

For the woman with a career outside the home, it may be the time she realises that she has gone about as far as she can go in her chosen work. The woman who has long harboured ideas of retraining may find that she is considered too old to train as a nurse or a teacher, despite having exactly the qualities and experience needed. We may have to come to terms with disappointments if they are not to sour us and get in the way of the many potential joys yet to come.

At this stage in life women, as 'the carers' in our society, often find themselves increasingly responsible for ageing parents. It is important that they do not become slaves to the elderly members of the family, any more than to the younger ones. There is a fine – but important – dividing line between being supportive and considerate and subjugating all of one's life to another. This is also a relevant point for those who look after children that are never going to be able to lead fully independent lives. It is important that women in this position seek and receive the utmost help in sorting out the future for themselves as well as their relatives. (See Useful Addresses for details of the Carers' National Association.) All these changes, or even just some of them, amount to life taking on a different direction and this can take quite a lot of mental adjustment.

With the prevalence of heart disease, cancer and other serious medical disorders, some women may find themselves widows during their late middle-age. Others suffer the galling experience of having the husband of many years, whose children they have raised and whose careers they have supported, desert them for another (usually younger) woman, sometimes even starting a new family. Nowadays, many people take early retirement, or are unfortunately made redundant. All these situations can be very demoralising and can determine to what extent the menopause will affect each individual. For this reason the menopause should not be underestimated by either those to whom it happens or her family and friends.

'Don't mind her, she is just being menopausal.' The very word 'menopausal' is all too often used to insult moody women. But these middle years often have a similar psychological effect on men. They, too, begin to realise the passage of time, that they are not immortal and that there are new 'facts of life' to be faced. The irritability, sleeplessness, indecision, aches and pains and sexual problems which are usually thought of as 'menopausal' are probably all general signs of ageing.

In the late twentieth century the message of the Western world is that in order to be beautiful it is necessary to be young. Isn't it therefore only logical to believe that to be old is to be ugly? Are signs of ageing any cause for dismay? No, that is clearly a waste of precious time. There are a great many plain young people around, and it is perfectly possible to be mature and attractive, even into advanced old age. I know a lady in Normandy who is now over 100 years old. She is single, her fiancé having been killed in the First World War. Now rather infirm, she spends her days sitting in her niece's kitchen corner in complete serenity, ready to talk politics, recipes, rave music, anything you choose. To be with her is to be made to feel interesting and that is the most attractive feature anyone can have. No, youth does not equal beauty any more than fertility is the same as femininity.

No mystery should surround the menopause. This is a moment to reorientate your life; to make sure that every moment is positive and constructive. The first thing to do is to rid ourselves of any annoying symptoms, exploring every avenue of help in doing so, and there are many which will be discussed in the following chapters. Then plans can be laid for a satisfying and exciting future.

———2———

The Symptoms and How to Deal With Them

Oestrogen is actually a group of hormones, produced in several parts of the body; not just the ovaries, but also the adrenal glands, skin and fatty tissue. Not only do they govern our sexuality, they have over 300 functions in maintaining the health of our skin, musculature, hair, digestion and brain. So it is not surprising that when they are unbalanced our whole being is in a highly sensitive and reactive state. In pre-menopausal women the main source of oestrogen is the kind that is produced by the ovaries. When this slackens off, we create a similar form of oestrogen from other hormones. Taking all this activity into account, it is no surprise that the menopause has an assortment of side-effects, and each one of us will have a different experience. As with hot flushes, it must be emphasised that the following depressing list is of 'possibles' not 'probables' which can all be helped, either with HRT, or other treatment.

Hot Flushes and Night Sweats

Although hot flushes are probably the best-known symptom of the menopause, they are not always the earliest. The first sign is quite often something out of the usual happening to the menstrual cycle. This may be irregular periods, happening more often or less often, or their being much lighter or much, much heavier, with clotting of the blood. But hot flushes are usually what first springs to mind when thinking about the menopause, because of their uncomfortable and uncontrollable nature.

Hot flushes and the associated night sweats are a symptom of the peri-menopausal phase. It seems that deficiency of the hormones involved in bringing on the menopause also have an effect on the way in which the body controls temperature. The body's thermostat becomes set too low, telling us that we are too cold. So the brain starts the mechanism for warming-up. This is done by expanding the blood vessels, allowing more blood to flow to the skin, causing it to redden and heat up. Often the brain then registers that it has overdone it and so switches on perspiration to cool down the overheated areas. This gives rise to anything from a slight clamminess to rivers of sweat.

Women who have hot flushes report everything from a sudden warm feeling to a sensation of tremendous heat and being bathed in perspiration. Even the mild, warm feeling is different from feeling ordinarily overheated as it is accompanied by a sudden increase in heart rate and blood pressure. This explains why, for some people, hot flushes cause anxiety and feelings of exhaustion.

Hot flushes and night sweats are extremely common but not every woman has them. Various surveys of women in mid-life have found that approximately three-quarters of them reported having hot flushes. While that means that a person is more likely to experience them than not, not everyone has the fiercest kind. It must, however be said that when flushing begins, it does usually get worse before it gets better, and that a very small minority continue to have flushes for many years. As with everything, it depends upon the individual.

It is an interesting fact that hot flushes do not occur in every society and they are generally more common in the west than in less developed countries. In our youth-worshipping society, we seem to have so many problems with middle age. Greek and Mayan women do not seem to be bothered by these symptoms.

However in Japan there is not even a word for hot flushes. In Greece, as in the Indian sub-continent, age is not dreaded and in Japan the elderly are venerated. In some countries where women are kept apart from general society during the fertile part of their lives, they can now come out into the world and experience a freedom they have not had since childhood.

Cultural differences aside, it is more likely that hot flushes and other symptoms are influenced by diet and life style. The Japanese diet is high in fish (which is a source of calcium) and soy, which has been found to contain oestrogen. Japanese women are also less 'motorised' than many Westerners, and the daily walk to the shops means regular exercise, helping to maintain a good circulation which is important for heat regulation. Thin women are more likely to have hot flushes than those who are slightly overweight, because fatty tissue is a source of oestrogen. These facts may be pointers to a way of coping with hot flushes and night sweats, even avoiding them altogether.

Hot flushes, although harmless to the health, can nevertheless be distressing. Perhaps the most important thing to remember when combatting the effects of a hot flush, however bad, is that it is never as obvious to onlookers as the sufferer thinks. Being afraid that you are making a spectacle of yourself can only aggravate matters, as you may become more hot and bothered and so will perspire more. It is helpful to keep a diary of both hot flushes and night sweats to see if a pattern develops. It then may be possible to avoid situations or foods that trigger them.

Keep your circulation and body in trim with regular, but non-stressful, exercise. Brisk walking is good for this, although other forms of exercise are necessary for the avoidance of other symptoms such as osteoporosis. This is because the hormones which protect our bones against osteoporosis are carried in the blood and the more they can get around to do their work the better. Keep your weight reasonable for your height. Aim to be neither too fat nor too thin. Take time to make sure you eat a good, balanced diet. It is all too easy for us to fall into bad nutritional habits, especially if we are not preparing regular healthy meals for a family.

Other things to avoid are living life in a rush, especially in hot weather. Do not hurry your meals and allow time for their digestion. Spicy foods, hot drinks, alcohol, sugar and caffeine (which is found in tea and chocolate as well as coffee) can all bring on attacks. Try to avoid overheated rooms and stressful situations. Smoking has a bad effect on the circulation and thus intensifies both hot flushes and night sweats, so this is another good reason for giving it up.

Wearing cotton clothing rather than nylon or polyester is a good move as cotton allows our skin to 'breathe' more and is cooler than artificial fibres. Silk is not such a good idea as perspiration marks it and becomes visible as wet patches very easily. Choose clothes without high necklines and with short sleeves. In cool weather, several layers of easily removable lightweight clothing are preferable to woollens, as it is easier to adjust if you feel a hot flush coming on. Keep a supply of cool drinks in a vacuum flask by you at work and one of those small hand-held battery-driven fans. Better still, have the central heating turned down. To persuade others to reduce the temperature, try suggesting it as an ecologically sound measure.

Cotton bed linen, too, is better than even a cotton/polyester mix in dealing with sweating at night. Night sweats can be severe and frequent and can be very disruptive to sleep, causing tiredness and consequent depression the following day. A movement of air in the bedroom, gained by opening both a window and door, can be helpful. A second hand-held battery fan kept beside the bed is useful, along with a bowl of tepid (not cold) water and a flannel for sponging down the face, neck and chest, will help. Allow the water to evaporate from the skin, rather than drying it, as this will greatly reduce the heat.

Hormone Replacement Therapy (HRT) has been found to be 98 percent effective in the elimination of both hot flushes and night sweats, but it is not suitable for everyone and some people initially prefer to try more natural medications, at first anyway (HRT will be discussed further in Chapter 4).

A visit to a qualified homoeopath or medical herbalist may produce just what is needed. At health-food shops, ginseng, dong quai, black cohosh and various other herbs and soya products, all of which contain oestrogen-like substances, may be bought over the counter. Sage is a traditional herb which is a rich source of natural oestrogen and can now be bought in tincture form for the express purpose of treating hot flushes. This and other herbs are worth a try under the guidance of a qualified medical herbalist. There are also herbal treatments for insomnia brought on by night sweats.

A course of acupuncture can also be beneficial. Learning techniques of relaxation and meditation are helpful in reducing stress and preparing for a good night's sleep, and can be used to good effect to reduce the worst of a hot flush when it comes.

Although neither hot flushes nor night sweats are a health hazard and much can be done to ease them, there may come a time when a visit to the doctor is indicated i.e. if sleep is so disturbed that it is impossible to get a good night's rest, or if hot flushes are seriously interfering with daily life or causing depression and exhaustion.

Two or three decades ago, tranquillisers would probably have been prescribed, with not too many questions asked. Now the situation should be much improved as GPs are more aware and understanding of the menopause and the psychological, as well as physical, effects that it has on many women. Now, thanks to the progress of medicine, women can be given Hormone Replacement Therapy (HRT). This delays the menopause and reduces its effects by supplying the body with the hormones that it ceases to produce on its own. HRT may not be prescribed as a matter of course and it is not without side-effects. There are various forms of HRT available and your doctor will be able to help you establish which one would be most suitable for you.

Incontinence

Surely nothing can induce the 'I must be getting old' feeling quite as much as finding you are unable to control your bladder. Incontinence can range from a slight spurt when you sneeze to truly wetting yourself if you are unable to get to a loo immediately when you first feel the need. These typify two different types of incontinence: stress incontinence and urge incontinence. Although hardly ever talked about, even among friends, both are very, very common and, fortunately, very treatable. For further information on incontinence, contact the Continence Foundation (see Useful Addresses).

STRESS INCONTINENCE

The muscles and tissues which support the bladder and its associated tubes become slackened with the passage of time due to childbearing, constipation, obesity and the general lessening of muscle tone caused by lack of oestrogen. A circular muscle is responsible for the opening and closing of the urethral openings through which urine leaves the body, and this and the other pelvic muscles can be strengthened by the frequent repetition of the kind of postnatal exercises new mothers are shown (see page 74). Ring pessaries of various designs are also available which will support internal organs that have sagged to the extent that they press or jog up and down on a full bladder when coughing, dancing or jumping. It may be worth talking to your GP about these. HRT will also help this kind of incontinence in the way that it helps all other kinds of musculature; with the oestrogen building-up muscle tone. Physiotherapy and surgery can also help.

URGE INCONTINENCE

With this type of incontinence, it is imperative for the sufferer to get to the lavatory the second he or she feels the need to. This is far from being a totally female complaint. It can be caused by infection, destruction of the nerves controlling the bladder or thinning of the tissues of the tubing along which the urine flows. The condition known as 'irritable bladder' is not fully understood. When the bladder is only partially full there is an irresistable urge to pass water as if the bladder were stretched to capacity. An infection, such as cystitis, can make the bladder overactive and medical advice should be sought to cure this.

In addition to medication, self-help is also possible, which is always a morale booster. Passing water is often very uncomfortable, even painful and it would seem that drinking lots of water would be the worst thing to do. In fact, this can be of considerable help in diluting the urine (strong urine stings more), and helping to wash out infecting bacteria. Drinking plenty of water also helps to combat stress incontinence as it helps to prevent the constipation that can weaken the pelvic muscles. Close fitting underwear of man-made materials also make for the warm, damp conditions that bacteria love, so loose cotton clothes are best. Tea and coffee are also best avoided as they are diuretics. Vaginal lubricants, such as acetic-acid jelly, will also alleviate the stinging as they counteract the alkaline environment in which infections develop. These are available from pharmacists.

Osteoporosis

Osteoporosis has been known about for many years. In old paintings ancient women, and some men too, are represented as bent and wizened, lame and leaning on sticks. Just because our bones seem solid and strong, we are tempted to think that they grow with their owners and once fully developed they are there to stay. To understand osteoporosis we have to understand our bones better than that.

Bone mass is constantly being broken down and remade and when we are still in the growth stage of life, the rebuilding of healthy bones is going on faster than the breaking-down side of the process. The cells that perform this function are also responsible for mending fractures. Eventually, with the passage of time, the breaking down takes place faster than the restructuring. This results in the weakening of the bone and allows fractures small and large to occur more easily. This is osteoporosis.

We have two sorts of bone: compact and spongy. The human skeleton is mostly composed of compact bone which takes time to weaken. The so-called spongy bone is different. It is not really spongy so much as constructed like a honeycomb. The solid surface is only a thin covering over a three-dimensional network of thin bone. It is this 'filling' that is most subject to degeneration. There is a good deal of this spongy filling in the top of the thigh bone, and in the vertebrae and wrist bones. Hence, it is at these points that breaks are most likely to occur.

Breaks can happen after even minor bumps which would only bruise or shake up a stronger person. This can result in a great deal of pain and disablement that can even be fatal. It has been found that 15 percent of all hip fractures result in the death of the sufferer through after-effects such as pneumonia and thrombosis.

It is very important to halt this thinning of our bones, although this can be difficult as the disease is unnoticeable in its early stages. Osteoporosis can start as early as the mid-thirties and its effects may pass unnoticed for a decade or so. The first symptoms are often back pain. If you cannot stand for as long as you want without developing back-ache, especially in the lower back, this can be a sign that the bones are thinning. Only later would the breaks and eventual deformity of the 'dowager's hump' occur, caused by crumbling of the vertebrae. So, osteoporosis is obviously something we all wish to avoid. There is plenty to be done beside resorting to HRT, which will be the answer for some.

Diet is important, especially calcium, as well as exercise. These are discussed in Chapters 5 and 6 respectively. Many of the rules for good eating hold true for good bone making. Alcohol, caffeine and nicotine are all culprits in preventing calcium from reaching its desired destination.

It may sound obvious, but get into the habit of making your home safe. Then everyone is less likely to have bone-cracking accidents in later life. Don't have loose rugs, highly polished floors or trailing flexes. Don't leave things on the stairs, but put them on a nearby table to prevent someone falling over them. Be especially careful around the house and outside if you are taking medicines which make you tired or light-headed. The National Osteoporosis Society can supply further information (see Useful Addresses).

Skin Problems

We tend to think of our skin as our outermost layer, but the most important part of it lies a few millimetres beneath the surface. The skin grows, replacing itself every few weeks, from this base layer and it is to this we need to pay the most attention. Applying creams and lotions is fun and can be soothing, healing and a great morale booster, but a good skin starts with good nutrition.

The skin and all internal organs are supported by material called connective tissue, a cross between padding and scaffolding which holds everything in place. Under a microscope, this looks like one of those modern pieces of weaving, thick and thin fibres of collagen and elastin mixed together, criss-crossing and forming an intricate mesh. Helping the skin in the continual process of renewal are the blood vessels, fat cells, hair follicles and nerve endings. Necessary to all this activity are the hormones and oxygen which are brought by the circulation of the blood. As early as our mid-thirties, this can all begin to slow up; the fat cells are reduced and the collagen and elastin become weaker, resulting in a number of effects.

The weakening of this support system and the reduction of its fat and moisture content causes the skin to wrinkle. The replacement of skin cells also slows down, so that the dead surface cells remain on the body for longer, becoming steadily drier through over-exposure to the elements. The condition of these surface cells reflects how healthy we really are or, more precisely, how our health was a few weeks ago when these cells were being formed.

But, depressing as this sounds, there is still much which can be done to improve things, even without HRT. Starting from the foundation of our skin, as with many other aspects of health, a healthy diet is the basic necessity. Make sure that the body receives all the nutrients it needs. Equally important is making sure that these nutrients are absorbed and utilised by the body effectively and this means keeping the blood circulation active. The right kind of exercise is necessary to boost circulation (see Chapter 6).

Smoking is a tremendous enemy of the more mature complexion. Not only does the side-stream of smoke make us screw up our eyes and increase wrinkling, smoking also reduces our circulation by narrowing the blood vessels, starving the skin of nutrition and suffocating it with lack of oxygen. Moderate consumption of red wine has recently been found to be beneficial in keeping the level of cholesterol in the blood low. But alcohol needs to be treated with caution, because it is dehydrating and, like smoking, constricts the blood vessels. The skin is under attack on several fronts in mid-life. The nerve endings can deteriorate with age and this can bring on a tickly itchiness, called formication.

When it comes to the effect of the weather on the skin, we tend to find ourselves in a *Catch 22* situation. The easiest way to obtain the vitamin D we need for healthy bones, is through exposure to the sun; but the trouble is that we have fewer melanocytes in our skins as we get older. These are the cells which contain protective pigment, melanin, which is released to protect us against the harmful UV rays of the sun by tanning our bodies. It is important to care for your skin from both outside and inside. Now that the relationship between exposure to UV rays and skin cancer is recognised, it is vital that we all wear a good sunscreen at all times, no matter what colour our skin is. Watch out for any sign of skin disorder and report it to the doctor at once. For a decade now the Australians in their hot climate have adopted the 'Slop, Slip, Slap' motto ... Slop on the sunscreen, Slip on a T-shirt, Slap on a hat. Fortunately, skin cancer is curable, provided that it is caught early enough. However, prevention is far better and although it is too late for us to undo the bad effects of three or four decades of unguarded sun-worship, we can start to protect our skin in the future. We can also help to educate the next generation – while a short time unprotected in the fresh air is good, we must treat the sun with caution.

Hair Problems

The reduced production of sebum which lubricates the skin has a similar effect on the hair. Our 'crowning glories' can become finer, limper, floppier and more difficult to style. The dry flakes which can appear on the face due to lack of sebum can crop up on the scalp too, so extra special hair care is necessary. The gentlest of shampoos are called for, used sparingly and diluted with warm water rather than poured on neat. Dry your hair as you would a tiny baby by patting gently instead of vigorous towelling. It may be worth trying a new style, perhaps spending the money on a wonderful cut rather than a drying perm. Don't be afraid to try something you might think 'too young'. Nothing is more ageing than the tight perm, especially on whitening hair.

An even less welcome, but fortunately much less likely problem, is that of hirsutism. When the production of oestrogen slackens the male hormones normally present in women get the upper hand. This can cause the fine hairs on the face, arms, legs and body to darken and coarsen. Fortunately, this responds well to low doses of HRT. The same condition can result in the lowering of the voice although this can also be a symptom of thyroid trouble and should be medically checked. There is a great deal which can be done to improve both skin and hair problems without having to resort to HRT.

Vaginal Dryness

The lessening of secretions affecting the visible areas is also at work unseen. A very vulnerable spot is the vagina and the area of skin immediately around it. The resulting dryness can make sexual intercourse uncomfortable and even painful and this often results in a reluctance to have sex. Unfortunately the effect of this is to cut off any supply of the natural lubrication which occurs during lovemaking. Not unnaturally, this can cause tension and depression which in turn inhibits the production of natural lubricants and the whole thing becomes a vicious circle.

This can be helped by the liberal use of lubricants (such as KY Jelly) which are sold over the counter at chemists and are now beginning to appear on the shelves of supermarkets. However, avoid creams containing petroleum jelly (such as Vaseline) if you are using condoms or a diaphragm for contraception, as this causes the latex to disintegrate.

Left unchecked, vaginal dryness can develop into a maddeningly itchy patch which, if scratched (the temptation is great), becomes raw and stings during urination. If this does not quickly improve, a trip to the doctor is indicated as these chronic raw patches can be treated successfully with non-hormonal medication.

While cleanliness is important, it is not a good idea to use a lot of soap, especially the perfumed kind, along with over-enthusiastic use of scented bath oils, talcum powders, shower gels and lotions. Another factor which aggravates the dryness is the use of the modern sanitary towel or tampon during either normal periods before the menopause or the induced bleed which is normal with HRT. These are now not only so efficient that you can 'Do a ten-hour aerobics class in your new white leotard without a second's worry', they also absorb every drop of the moisture that this area of your poor body is trying to lubricate itself with. The answer to this is to cover the area well with a lubricating cream.

Breast Problems

Just as a woman's breasts develop during the hormonal changes of puberty, they change again during the menopause. Oestrogen depletion causes weakening of the supporting tissues of the whole body and so the breasts tend to sag under their own weight. HRT can correct this to a certain extent but exercises such as those described in Chapter 6, will also help.

The commonest breast problems are mastalgia and mastitis. Mastalgia is the condition where breasts become hard and painful, sometimes extremely so. This appears to be an extension of the breast tenderness many women experience before a period. One of the causes can be too high a dose of oestrogen during Hormone Replacement Therapy; if so this can be adjusted. Another cause may be that the body has low levels of essential fatty acids and here a daily dose of evening primrose oil may help (see my *Quick Guide to Evening Primrose Oil*). Obtaining a really well-fitting bra and even wearing it at night may also help to ease the discomfort.

Mastitis, on the other hand, is a condition where the breasts become lumpy due to fibrous tissue forming knotted lumps or cysts. The effect has been described as the breasts feeling like a pair of old flock pillows! Many women develop these fibrocystic lumps in their late thirties and forties and the onset of the menopause actually diminishes them.

Another type of breast cyst is formed by fluid being retained in the tissues and forming smooth, movable lumps.

None of these conditions are life-threatening, which is probably why they have not attracted a great deal of attention from the medical researchers. One factor that has become apparent is that caffeine aggravates the situation. When this was eliminated from the diet of a sample of sufferers, 65 percent reported a great improvement in the condition of their breasts. This rose to 85 percent when evening primrose oil was taken as well. Sometimes these benign lumps are also treated satisfactorily with an externally applied progesterone cream.

Naturally when any breast lumps are discovered there is the fear that they might be cancerous. Any lump should be reported without delay to the doctor. The same goes for any change in shape or position of the breast, any dimpling, or discharge from the nipple, any lumps in the armpit or collarbone area or any swelling of the upper arm. Only one in ten lumps is discovered to be malignant (cancerous), but it is *essential* for these to be dealt with early. No GP will think that you are making a fuss if you present him or her with any of these symptoms. The organisation Women's Health can help with all women's health problems (see Useful Addresses).

Body Shape

Middle-aged spread is also associated with the menopause, although this is not truly a menopausal symptom as it seems to affect men as much as it does women. As the years go by our metabolic rate naturally slows down. To keep to more or less the same weight we need to eat fewer calories, preferably accompanied by more exercise. Unfortunately, our appetite often stays the same and our inclination to go out to the gym on cold, wet evenings usually diminishes.

Although we need fewer calories, our nutritional requirements of vitamins, minerals, etc remains. This makes it especially important not to fill ourselves up with the 'empty calories' of sugar and highly refined processed foods. By far the largest part of our food intake should be nutritious.

One reason for the thickening waistline in older women is the result of the shortening of the spine brought on by osteoporosis (see above). If overall height is reduced, but the weight remains the same, the poundage has to go somewhere and if it can't go up it must go out. Taking care to remember good posture can help to make you look slimmer than you are. Figure problems are dealt with in greater detail in Chapters 5 and 6.

Depression

Lastly, true clinical depression is not found any more frequently in middle-aged women than in any other age group. While this means that some menopausal women will be technically 'depressed', there are many more who will recognise in themselves, and be depressed by, several of the other symptoms in the above list. Thankfully, the majority of these symptoms can be relieved to a great extent if the oestrogen levels in the system are kept sufficiently high.

Oestrogen is involved in so many of our bodies' functions, both mental and physical, it is hardly surprising that it is hailed as a cure-all. It is only when we experience something as dramatic as the menopause that we realise just how important is the role hormones play. During the menopause, many women suddenly feel as though they have been stripped of their femininity and sexuality and this can be very depressing. However, this unpleasant symptom can almost always be rectified by maintaining our levels of oestrogen. There are many different medical views on the best way of increasing oestrogen levels. It can be done artificially with Hormone Replacement Therapy in one of its many forms (see Chapter 4). There are also alternative methods of bumping up the quantity of this all-important substance, such as increasing your intake of herbs that are rich in oestrogen (see page 21).

There are other reasons for the mental disorders which raise their heads in the middle years. These are quite often corrected by proper nutrition which is discussed in more detail in Chapter 5. Exercise is often effective in relieving anxiety and depression as it has been found to release chemicals from the brain into the blood supply and these induce a 'feel-good' factor (see Chapter 6).

It must be said, though, that if anyone, middle aged or not, is feeling that life is not worth living to the extent that they consider suicide, help should be sought at once, either from a GP or the Samaritans (their main London number is 0171-734 2800 and local numbers are in telephone directories).

3

Surgical Choices

There are a number of conditions, which turn up at the time of the menopause, that are not necessarily caused by it. Some of these are more serious than others and all require medical attention.

Gynaecological Problems

One of the most common afflictions of middle-aged women are fibroids. These are lumps of tissue inside the uterus which become knotted and fibrous. They are not cancerous or dangerous, but they can be the source of much discomfort. Apart from causing swelling, which can be considerable, they also trigger bleeding, which is not only a nuisance, but can be a cause of anaemia (iron deficiency). It is sometimes possible to remove fibroids without having to remove the uterus.

It is very important to report any irregular bleeding to the doctor, whether it is heavy or spotting.

If the uterus is found to be cancerous, a hysterectomy is likely. A total hysterectomy involves the removal of the uterus and the cervix, the neck of the womb. A partial or sub-total hysterectomy is the removal of only part of the uterus. Sometimes the ovaries are removed as well. This is called an oophorectomy, a bilateral oophorectomy being the removal of both ovaries. The fallopian tubes can also be removed.

Ovaries are, of course, removed if they are cancerous. Ovarian cancer is one of the most difficult forms of cancer to diagnose and surprisingly it is a bigger killer than AIDS. The charity called Research into Ovarian Cancer (ROC; see Useful Addresses) was set up in 1993. It funds research into the causes of ovarian cancer and investigates various treatments of this disease. Ovarian cancer usually occurs in young women. However, it can sometimes be detected in older women by appearing to be a very early menopause. It is known as the silent killer, as it is often only detected when it has reached an advanced and, unfortunately, fatal stage. Often, cancer of the ovaries is discovered during another operation, such as a partial hysterectomy. If this is the case, the ovaries will almost certainly be removed at the same time.

If a woman needs a hysterectomy, her ovaries are usually left intact. If they are removed, oestrogen production stops dead, menopausal symptoms start very suddenly and Hormone Replacement Therapy has to begin at once to counteract this. Because there is no uterus for excess lining material to build up in, the secondary hormone, progesterone, whose job it is to remove it, is no longer needed, so this hormone does not need to be replaced.

In post-menopausal women, or women about to become so, a surgeon will sometimes suggest that while undergoing a necessary hysterectomy, the ovaries are removed as well. In the case of uterine cancer, the ovaries are removed to limit the production of oestrogen as this hormone feeds this particular cancer. This is especially true for those women who have a family history of ovarian cancer. If there is other evidence of diseased ovaries, cysts for example, this indicates that removal of the ovaries would be a good idea. If, however, the ovaries are still perfectly healthy, it is a matter of debate whether their removal would be the right course of action and the issue should be discussed thoroughly by the surgeon and his or her patient before any operation. Make sure that you discuss all the options with your surgeon *before* being operated on. If there is any procedure that you do not want carried out, or any organ that you do not want removed, it is important to make this clear both verbally and also in writing on the surgery consent form that you will be asked to sign.

Any hysterectomy is major surgery in a particularly delicate and intricate part of the body. There are many other bodily functions which could be badly affected as a result of the operation. Add to this the risk that any operation on the body cavity can induce post-operative fever and infection, and it becomes clear that a hysterectomy is not to be undertaken lightly. If the operation is to save your life, then the decision is easy to make. If it is to relieve symptoms such as pain and haemorrhage, it is worth exploring every other avenue of treatment first. The best person to advise you is your GP, whose mind does not automatically run along the lines of surgery – even if your GP does advise surgery, you can ask for a second opinion.

Much has been written about the importance of regular cervical smears. These enable the signs of cervical cancer to be detected so that any further development of the cancer can be stopped. Even after a hysterectomy in which the cervix is removed, it is important to continue with smear tests as the top of the vagina is where cancer is likely to recur. This test is also useful for detecting other diseases of the vagina.

Endometriosis is another problem which only affects women. About 10–15 percent of women between the ages of twenty-five and forty-five have this condition. It has been known about for well over a century but is still something of a medical mystery. Endometrial tissue should only line the uterus in preparation of receiving a fertilised egg and if this does not occur it breaks up and is shed in the normal menstrual blood flow. It can, however, escape and appear outside the uterus, turning up almost anywhere in the pelvic cavity. It tries to follow the monthly pattern and bleeds during menstruation. This may not only cause pain, but when it heals, scar tissue is formed and this can build up month after month. The offending tissue then presses on other organs and causes more pain, possible infertility and ovarian cysts. Diagnosis is difficult. It does not always cause pain and the pain may have other causes.

Endometriosis can be very difficult to treat. Various forms of male hormone treatment are tried but side-effects can be unpleasant and the long-term effects are not yet known. Surgery is a possibility but the problem tissue is difficult to locate. Sometimes treatment is tried by laser or cauterisation. Many surgeons are only in favour of treating the disease itself if it is a cause of infertility which the woman wants reversed. Otherwise the pain sometimes responds to the contraceptive pill or anti-inflammatory drugs. Evening primrose oil and the B vitamins may be of help, otherwise the only suggestion is painkillers. If all this sounds very negative, the one cheering aspect is that the menopause often brings an end to the problem. The Endometriosis Society is a self-help group for sufferers (see Useful Addresses).

Another very painful condition with symptoms which can be confused with endometriosis is pelvic inflammatory disease. Unlike endometriosis, this is a very serious condition which can prove fatal. It is usually, though not always, sexually transmitted. In contrast, endometriosis is not life threatening and is more often suffered by the celibate woman.

Non-cancerous conditions which are sometimes treated by surgery in middle age include the various forms of prolapse. Badly managed childbirth, ageing, obesity, lack of oestrogen, strenuous athleticism, constipation and even prolonged coughing fits, can all cause the 'hammock' of pelvic muscle to sag. Instead of supporting the uterus and bladder, it weakens and the organs slip downwards. The uterus falls into the vagina and in extreme cases can finish up outside the body. The bladder can fall backwards or the rectum bulge forwards to press into the wall of the vagina. Any of these displacements causes varying degrees of discomfort and if the exercises (such as those described in Chapter 6) are ineffective, and the prolapse is too bad to be held in place with a ring pessary, surgery may be necessary.

Breast Problems

Although the vast majority of all breast lumps are benign and do not cause a problem, the question of mastectomy – a breast removal – arises in cases where cancerous tissue is found. When any cancer is found, Hormone Replacement Treatment is automatically stopped as cancer cells feed on oestrogen.

A mastectomy varies enormously depending upon the extent of the cancer. The worst possibility is the radical mastectomy. This removes the affected breast, all its underlying muscles and all the associated lymph nodes in the armpit on that side of the body. The lymph nodes are part of the body's defence system but in acting against cancer cells they very often become affected themselves and are known as secondary sites for cancer. Sometimes there is an argument for performing this type of drastic surgery with the thought that it might well remove the need for another operation later on. General anaesthetics and opening up the body are always best kept to a minimum.

Fortunately, the more usual form is the modified radical mastectomy, which involves less of the musculature and fewer lymph nodes being removed. Becoming more common, probably because of earlier diagnosis, is the quadrantectomy. This is when only a quarter of the breast, where the lump is, is removed. Even better is the lumpectomy, where only the lump itself is taken. Sometimes this operation is accompanied by implanting the radioactive element iridium. The radioactivity wears off in a matter of weeks, forming a course of internal radiotherapy.

Non-surgical options include two types of chemotherapy; one for the kind of breast cancer which is associated with oestrogen and another for the kind that is not. The first has fewer side-effects. As with a hysterectomy, if you are unlucky enough to be in this position, this is something which needs careful discussion with your doctor, your surgeon, your family and friends and possibly one of the associations set up to give such advice. The Women's Nationwide Cancer Control Campaign and Breast Cancer Care are two such organisations (see Useful Addresses). Even today, surgeons are predominantly male and cannot be expected always to understand the sense of violation a woman can experience at losing one of her most feminine features.

It may seem strange but it is true of all cancers that the older you are when it develops, the better are the chances of recovery. In a young body, especially in a child, all the cells are dividing, developing and growing at a tremendous rate. This goes for cancerous cells as well as those that are healthy. The key to any form of successful cancer treatment is an early diagnosis. All women, no matter what their age, must examine their breasts regularly for lumps and have regular cervical smear tests.

4

Hormone Replacement Therapy

So much research is being carried out on Hormone Replacement Therapy (HRT) that new facts are being discovered almost daily. The result is that there is a huge amount of often conflicting advice bombarding women from every side. It doesn't help that many GPs are almost as bewildered as the rest of us. Visit a menopause clinic or well women centre if you are thinking of giving HRT a try. Organisations such as the Marie Stopes Centre and the Margaret Pyke Centre – see Useful Addresses – can assess suitability for HRT and offer advice.

Many, many women try HRT, for a great variety of reasons, but a huge number give up within the first year of what could be a long and profitable treatment. Their GPs naturally start them on one of the standard prescriptions and if it proves to be unsatisfactory it is all too easy to get the feeling that 'we've tried that but it didn't work'. However, the initial prescription can be just the first step in quite a complicated process of trial and adjustment of type and dosage until the most suitable is found. In addition, research is continually turning up new possibilities so the permutations are almost endless.

Hormone Replacement Therapy was first used in the 1950s for the treatment of hot flushes. The long-term benefits of the therapy gradually became apparent over the next twenty years when it was found that the women so treated were less subject to osteoporosis and heart disease. Thus it began to be used directly for these purposes. It will be many years before it is proved that taking HRT is good for the heart by being prescribed primarily for this purpose, but so far it does seem that this may be the case.

In the 1960s, HRT began to be associated less happily with the health of the womb. The form of HRT used was of oestrogen only which causes a thickening of the lining of the womb, such as happens in the first part of the menstrual cycle. Unlike the natural cycle, the lining is not shed, but builds up, causing the condition called hyperplasia which is associated with cancer of the uterus. To counteract this, progesterone is prescribed, causing the thickened lining to be shed monthly, imitating the menstrual period. It has been found that the amount of progesterone given is not as important as the length of time for which it is taken. This is what is called opposed therapy, the oestrogen and progesterone apparently 'opposing' one another in the building up and then the shedding of the lining of the womb. If oestrogen alone is taken, there is a 7–15 percent increase in this hyperplasia which reduces to nil if progesterone is taken for a period of twelve days.

Most people take HRT because they want relief from uncomfortable symptoms although it is also a good countermeasure against osteoporosis, which can begin several years before periods stop or hot flushes begin. HRT is automatically part of the treatment when a woman has her ovaries removed, otherwise menopausal symptoms set in with a vengeance.

Taking HRT reduces the risk of heart disease which is much less common in young women than in post-menopausal women. When oestrogen levels fall at the peri-menopause, women are subject to heart trouble to the same extent as men. There seems to be no upper age limit for the start of treatment by HRT but the thought of restarting monthly bleeds after perhaps years of freedom may be unattractive. One of the main side-effects can be a very heavy induced monthly bleed. This can be cured by an adjustment of the dosage which may take some trial and error but is well worth the trouble. Also in many cases the 'false menstruation' becomes lighter as time goes by. Another combination is being researched which, although combining both oestrogen and progesterone in opposition, is small enough in dosage to result in no bleeding, even from the first month. This is obviously ideal. A few people, less than 5 percent, find that they are intolerant to all forms of HRT.

How to Take HRT

There are many types of HRT treatment. The commonest, in the United Kingdom and America at least, is the oral form, and the commonest form of this is the 'calendar pack' sort. This arrives on a neat little bubblepack card, so it is quite clear what is to be taken and when. There is an oestrogen pill for every day and a progesterone one to be taken for twelve of those days. All very straightforward and wonderful if it works. The trouble is we are all individuals and what suits one person will upset another. The right dose for one person is too much or not enough for another.

One adverse symptom can be nausea, which may or may not pass off of its own accord. It is tempting to think of HRT as simply replicating the normal menstrual cycle but this is not quite the case. Before the menopause the ovaries release hormones straight into the bloodstream. If they are taken by mouth, in order to reach the bloodstream they have to go through the digestive system, including the liver, which could account for the nausea. Taking a pill is flexible in that treatment can be stopped at any time, but the dose of hormone is released suddenly into the system, causing digestive upsets.

A suitable alternative may be wearing a patch. These are like pieces of sticking plaster each carrying a dose of hormones in alcohol. This way the hormones are released into the body gradually through the skin, by-passing the digestive system and any of these disadvantages. The patches have to be changed every few days and originally, progesterone pills had to be taken to have the necessary opposition to the oestrogen. Now there is a patch available which combines the two hormones in suitable dosage, another example of the continuing research working towards the perfecting of this therapy. The patches are worn on any fleshy part of the lower body. Some people develop an allergic reaction to the adhesive or the alcohol in the patch, although there are various ways of overcoming this. The patch form of treatment appears to have all the good effects of the oral variety. However, it has not been in use long enough to prove that it has all the beneficial long-term effects.

Both the oral variety of HRT and the patch form are treatments which involve remembering to use them properly day by day. An implant avoids this and is particularly suitable for women who have undergone a hysterectomy and who, because they have no womb to be 'over lined', do not need the opposing pills of progesterone. After the tiny pellet has been placed under the skin, often in a GP's surgery under local anaesthetic, it can be forgotten about until menopausal symptoms return and it needs replacing. This can be after as much as six months, but some women find that the replacing has to be done at ever-decreasing intervals. The return of menopausal symptoms seems to indicate that the effect of the implant has worn off, but sometimes these symptoms, which are caused by a fall in oestrogen level, are accompanied by breast tenderness and other symptoms of too high an oestrogen level. If this is experienced it would be advisable to transfer to another form of HRT.

It is never a good idea, whatever form is used, to stop treatment suddenly – some symptoms, particularly hot flushes and night sweats, are brought on by falling oestrogen levels rather than simply a low level. As an implant is almost impossible to remove it is obviously not suitable for someone trying out HRT for the first time. However, it can be a very successful treatment for someone who is a proven suitable subject. Like the patch the hormone is absorbed straight into the blood, avoiding the liver. It has the added advantage that testosterone can be used with it. This is generally thought of as a male hormone but is also present in women in very small quantities. Lack of it can cause a loss of interest in sex, great tiredness and lack of confidence. Testosterone cannot be given orally as it could harm the liver.

There are also skin and vaginal creams and pessaries. These are useful for women who have problems with vaginal dryness, itching and problems passing urine, though they are not strong enough to cure any other symptoms or prevent bone loss.

The Cancer Question

HRT has long been suspected of increasing the risk of various cancers. The increased risk of developing uterine cancer used to be great, but that was before the 'opposed' type of dosage was used. Now that a monthly bleed removes the build-up of the uterine lining the risk of cancer of the womb is the same for women on HRT as it is for anyone else. Other female cancers, of the ovaries and the cervix, are also apparently unaffected by the use of HRT.

Many factors are involved and are taken into consideration when a woman thinks of starting HRT treatment; for example, if breast cancer runs in her family, or if she has suffered disorders of the breast in the form of benign lumps, the presence of which would make malignant lumps harder to detect. If she did not undergo the menopause until her mid-fifties or is obese, doctors are reluctant to prescribe HRT in any form. Some breast cancers seem associated with the production of oestrogen and if the body has already been high in that hormone then it would seem unwise to give it more.

Statistics show that one in twelve women will develop breast cancer. There seems no doubt in scientists' minds that there is no increased risk of the development of breast cancer if HRT is taken for less than five years; the risk does increase slightly after this. Having come to terms with that, we also have to remember that in post-menopausal women heart disease and stroke are far bigger killers than breast cancer. HRT has been found to decrease heart problems and to reduce the number of strokes more than it increases the risk of breast cancer. (Contact the British Heart Foundation for further preventative information – see Useful Addresses.) Bear in mind also that women receiving HRT are under close medical supervision and would receive immediate attention should the worst happen.

Conclusions of one study, conducted in 1993 by the consultant gynaecologist Dr John Studd and associates and published in the *British Journal of Hospital Medicine*, are as follows:

* The oestrogen in HRT improves depression.
* HRT has not been prescribed primarily to help heart conditions, so it is not possible to say that it should be. However, it does seem that people who take HRT are less likely to suffer heart problems.
* As the hormone content of HRT is not the same as that of the contraceptive pill, there is no reason to think that people with a history of thrombosis should not take it.
* HRT prevents the acceleration of bone loss and acts to increase its density. Taking HRT results in a 30 percent increase in skin thickness with a 34 percent increase in the amount of collagen.
* There is no major increase in the risk of breast cancer and what there is, is balanced out by a corresponding decrease in the death rate from this disease.
* Unopposed HRT is a possibility for women suffering from osteoporosis who do not want a monthly bleed.

They should be aware of the possibility of endometrial (uterine) cancer and have regular checks for it.

* Not only gynaecologists should think of using HRT for their patients but also heart specialists, psychiatrists and neurologists.

Some say that they do not wish to go in for HRT because they feel that it is unnatural. This could be said also of wearing glasses, having a heart pacemaker or taking antibiotics. We are not really designed to last as long as we do. Zoologically speaking we are supposed to reproduce ourselves and then there is no further need for our survival so, as women, anything we do to prolong our lives after the menopause is unnatural. Unfairly, this point is reached far sooner by women than men, whose reproductive lives are much longer. The physical strain of their part in the reproductive cycle is much less than it is for the female of the species!

The Alternatives to HRT

So far there is no direct alternative to conventional HRT. However, homoeopaths can offer many avenues of treatment to try. If you and your doctor come to the conclusion that HRT is not for you, then homoeopathy may well be the answer. There is a small but steadily increasing band of conventionally trained GPs with a postgraduate qualification in homoeopathy. Becoming a patient of such a doctor is the ideal for homoeopathic treatment for any condition. The next best alternative is to find a qualified lay homoeopath (see Useful Addresses).

Acupuncture, aromatherapy, reflexology, Chinese medicine, herbalism, cranial osteopathy, shiatsu and yoga all have their part to play but it is impossible to generalise. All these methods are individually tailored to the patient's needs and a great deal depends upon the skill of the practitioner, so it is very important to go to a qualified practitioner (see Useful Addresses).

Diet is extremely important too, as oestrogen is also found in plant form. As has been said, the Japanese style of eating contains a great deal of natural oestrogen in the form of soya products and oily fish. In *The Silent Passage*, the American writer Gail Sheehy quotes Dr Serafina Corsello who has thoroughly studied herbal remedies for menopausal symptoms at her nutritional centre in New York. Her findings are that the Chinese herb, dong quai, contains a good deal more oestrogen than Premarin, which is the drug form most used conventionally. Other oestrogen-rich herbs are mentioned on page 21. It is advisable, as with all treatments, to take expert advice as to dosage, etc; contact the National Institute of Medical Herbalists (see Useful Addresses).

Useful books for further reading on the menopause and HRT are listed at the end of this *Quick Guide*.

5

Foods for Health

The Duchess of Windsor once said, 'we can never be too rich or too thin'. Wealth and how to acquire it is beyond the scope of this *Quick Guide*, but how about the much discussed subject of weight? Regardless of what the fashion magazines would have us believe, it *is* possible to be medically underweight. The underweight are more likely to suffer from hot flushes, early menopause, tiredness and reduced immunity to infections. Research has also shown that the underweight amongst the elderly are likely to die before the plump. As a group, Westerners are often accused of being overweight, but it is now found that almost 90 percent of the female members try to lose weight at some point to the extent that they feel hungry, cold, tired and perpetually preoccupied with food. This is no basis for living a full life.

There is also no excuse for going around looking like a bladder of lard. The lack of collagen brought on by low oestrogen production has a bad effect on the overall structure of the body, the bones and muscles, as well as on the plumpness and resilience of the skin. As our bones and muscles are what we move about with, we must try to keep them in as good a condition as possible for as long as possible in order to keep mobile. Fortunately there is a great deal we can do in this respect to keep ourselves flexible and active, and our internal organs unencumbered with the burden of excess fat. The younger we all start it the better. Provided that you were in good shape at twenty there is no harm in being a stone heavier at fifty. How you feel and the shape you are in is what matters. If when you look in the mirror you seem to see the word FAT above your head, cross out the A, substitute an I and make FIT your aim from now on.

First of all there is the old saying, 'we are what we eat'. Everything we take in through our mouths is processed by the body into the materials it needs. Food is turned into such necessaries as bone and teeth, muscle, blood or brain cells and nerves. Even our hormones are constructed originally from the food we eat. Our bodies can only be as good as the materials we supply and good nourishment is as important now as in pregnancy if we are to make the most of life. One of the big hurdles to overcome is the feeling that if we eat well but do not keep the calories down as much as possible we shall blow up like balloons.

The basic essentials are good nutrition and suitable exercise, both in sufficient quantity. Both of these can help avoid problems of heart trouble, angina, blood pressure, circulation, varicose veins, incontinence and a host of other ailments. So they really are worth taking trouble over!

Keeping in good shape can begin with exactly that. There is now a ratio between the size of your waist and hips which it is important to aim for. Take your relaxed waist measurement at its smallest and your hip measurement at its widest. Divide the waist by the hips. If the answer is 0.8 or a little less, that is ideal. If it is more, it is time to take steps. So a person with a 32" waist and 43" hips is just in the clear. However, if a basically petite woman with 36" hips also has a 32" waist she is just over the desired ratio. The presence of too much internal fat is very important to health. It puts a strain on all our internal organs, heart, lungs, liver, bladder, uterus, the lot.

Slimming

There are scores of books written on the subject of dieting, including my *Quick Guide to Successful Slimming*. Crash diets are really not a good idea for permanent weight loss. They nearly always end up with the lost weight being put back on quite quickly and a little more besides. This stretches an already weakened skin causing sagging – not a happy thought.

If you have only a few pounds to lose here are a few measures which could just do the trick for you in only a few weeks.

* Drink a large glass of water before each meal. Most of us do not drink enough plain water anyway. It is good for the complexion as well as the figure. If you have not done this before, a tumblerful of water can look a little daunting, but you may be surprised how soon your system will get used to it and you will actually look forward to it.
* Use a smaller plate than usual to prevent yourself taking more than you need.
* Eat as slowly as you can, sitting quietly and enjoying every forkful.
* Resist second helpings.
* Follow the saying 'Eat like a king at breakfast, a duke at noon and a pauper for the rest of the day'. That way your body has the best chance of burning off the calories eaten.
* Keeping a diary of eating can prove revealing. Write down everything eaten, when it was eaten and why, for reasons of hunger, sociability, tiredness, depression, to get warm. Only the first is a reason, the rest are excuses!
* When you are hungry, don't plan menus, shop for food or cook.
* Although we have all been brought up to eat three meals a day with no snacking in between, it may be helpful to eat the same amount each day but split into six smaller meals. This will keep your blood sugar level

up and so stop feelings of sudden hunger and tiredness, and consequent overeating, when meal times come around again.

* Cut out fatty and fried foods and switch to low-fat alternatives.

If the number of pounds you need to lose is in double figures you may need to take stronger measures. Different ways of weight loss suit different people. Food combining, where basically you eat what you like and in whatever quantity as long as you do not mix proteins and carbohydrates at a sitting and eat fruit only at certain times of day is a well-proven method. This is quite a complex system and needs to be studied from a specialist book on the subject (yes, there is a *Quick Guide to Food Combining*).

Joining a slimming club can be supportive. These range from the simple calorie counting and comparing of notes with others over a cup of (black!) tea, to the internationally known Weight Watchers (see Useful Addresses), which teaches a complete programme of healthy eating.

Nutrition Guidelines

Weight control is by no means the only aspect of nourishment to be revised at mid-life. Good nutrition is especially important if we are to get as much as possible out of life and this is the main object of this book.

We need calcium for our muscles and for the clotting of blood. Some women complain of bleeding of the gums and skin cuts being slow to heal. This could be due to a lack of calcium in the body. The calcium taken by the blood for clotting after injury could also be a cause of calcium depletion in the bones.

A few years ago there was a famous advertising slogan which exhorted us all to 'Drinka-pinta-milka-day'. This does go a great way to supplying the body's calcium needs but, in its full-fat form, milk is bad for cholesterol levels. Turning to at least semi-skimmed, if not fat-free, milk would take care of this. However, a pint of milk takes quite a bit of getting through unless you are really keen on it; if you do find this difficult another possibility is to use dried skimmed milk powder made up to double strength.

Try to find organically produced milk, especially in its skimmed, or at least semi-skimmed form. If dairy cows are dosed with medication this passes not only into their meat but also their milk, and on to us. Fat-soluble pesticides can turn up in milk, butter and cream. It may be easier to find organic goat's milk than cow's milk. Soya milk is good for people with allergies, but choose calcium-enriched varieties as ordinary soya milk contains little of this important mineral.

If you find milk indigestible, it may be more easily taken in the form of low-fat yoghurt. Infusing cardamom seeds in milk is said to make it more digestible and less mucus-forming (it also has the reputation of being a powerful ingredient in love potions!). Vegans drink no milk at all and have to go to very careful lengths to get enough calcium.

Hard and full-fat cream cheeses are best kept to a minimum because of the large amounts of fat they contain. Fortunately for cheese lovers there are cheeses now being made with much of the fat removed. Low-fat cottage cheese is available with all sorts of added natural flavours. It is also possible to make up your own favourites with fresh herbs.

Margarine is often bought as a healthier substitute for butter but the hydrogenation of the oils in it takes away much of the advantages it has over butter on the health front. Read the small print on the packaging to see what you are buying. This goes for everything bought in a packet.

Green vegetables such as broccoli are a good source of calcium, as is blackstrap molasses. Oily fish such as salmon and sardines are useful too, although you must eat the bones as well to obtain enough calcium. Stock made from well-boiled meat or fish bones and used in cooking is also a good way of getting calcium into the diet.

Tofu, a product made from soya and now becoming more and more readily available, is a very useful food to incorporate into any diet for many reasons beside its calcium content. Tofu is an extremely useful source of protein which is made from soya. On its own it is bland but this makes it very easy to flavour. There are now cookery books devoted to the preparation of meals using tofu, which has the advantage of being cheap as well as nourishing.

In previous generations, providing 'good red meat' on a daily basis was every housewife's aim for her family. Now we are beginning to see that red meat is not so desirable after all. As the quantity available has increased, the quality has decreased. This is a result of factory farming where beasts are fed growth hormones and antibiotics. These do not magically disappear in the slaughterhouse but travel with the carcase to the butcher's block and onto our plates. It is also found that we can become hardened to the effects of antibiotics if we take them too often. If we are dosed with them in the food we eat, we could find that when we need them for ourselves they are ineffective. Antibiotics, while they have their place in the medical armoury, also have less desirable effects. They encourage vaginal thrush by killing good bacteria as well as disease-causing ones, and leave many people with depression. Both these are something a middle-aged woman can well do without. Fortunately there are more and more organic farms and butcher's shops. Organically produced meat is even finding its way onto the supermarket shelves.

Results of studies on vegetarian women in America have found that red meat seems to leach calcium from the body, weakening the bones. Naturally it is more expensive to produce meat organically, but with the consumption of red meat limited to only once or twice a week and supplemented with tofu, the protein budget should remain the same.

Even the best red meats contain some saturated fat. A balanced diet should contain a little saturated fat, 10 percent (instead of the more usual 50+ percent found in a typical Western diet) and perhaps twice as much unsaturated fat in the form of vegetable oils. These contain essential fatty acids, so called because we need them but our bodies cannot make them. These are found in oily fish and in nut and seed oils such as olive oil. These oils should be used cold as dressing and not cooked which tends to destroy their goodness. The linoleic acid which is found in vegetable oils needs to be converted by the body to gamma-linoleic acid, GLA, and this conversion can be blocked by smoking, alcohol, air pollution, and lack of certain vitamins and minerals. In this case, a short cut is to take the GLA itself in the form of evening primrose oil capsules.

A large amount of fat is to be avoided because it not only encourages us to put on fat of our own, it seems to have links with the development of breast cancer.

Meat products, such as corned beef and sausages by their nature contain large amounts of fat. They also contain much more sodium than potassium. While people suffering from high blood pressure are rightly advised to cut out salt because of the sodium it contains, it now appears that it is also important to keep up the proportion of potassium to sodium in the system. The more processed and refined a food is, the more the potassium content goes down and the sodium goes up. Beside processed meat products, other foods which contain far greater proportions of sodium to potassium and should be avoided on this account are white bread, smoked fish and tinned vegetables. For this reason if for no other it is wise to stick to fresh organic red meat in small amounts, wholewheat flour, unsmoked foods and fresh vegetables.

Processed cereal packets have to be carefully read as they often contain huge quantities of sugar. Home-made muesli is best as you know what is in it and can make it to your own taste. Much cereal is eaten for its fibre content, which is good for avoiding diverticulitis and intestinal cancer, but raw or lightly cooked vegetables contain a great deal of fibre and if eaten in sufficient quantities can provide all the body's needs.

In lands where longevity is common, the diet tends to rely heavily on fresh fruit, raw vegetables, nuts and seeds for oils with very little meat or dairy products. This must prove something!

When it comes to nutrition, one thing we can all be certain of is that there are three S's we can all do without, male or female, menopausal or not:

* Sugar from the sugar basin
* Salt in cooking or on the table
* SMOKING!

SUGAR

There are claims that sugar is a natural substance and is necessary for energy. Sugar is indeed a plentiful source of calories but these are 'empty' calories, bringing nothing with them in the shape of nutritional value. How nutritional is sugar? So lacking that not even germs or moulds will live on it. The energy released by eating sugar is short-lived and is followed by a great dip in energy levels. The younger body is able to work through these highs and lows in the blood sugar level but it is an unwarranted strain on our glands as time passes.

Eating refined sugar can cause the body to be deficient in the B vitamins. This deficiency leads to tiredness and depression and links have been found between a lack of the B vitamins and the form of breast cancer which is associated with oestrogen imbalance. As research into athletic sports has shown, it is much better to give your body the more 'slow release' energy of unrefined carbohydrates. This is the kind found in wholemeal bread, pasta, brown rice and potatoes with their skins on. The digestion of sugar causes stress to the digestive system and it has been suggested that it may block the absorption of calcium needed to avoid osteoporosis.

It may be revealing to make a note of how much sugar you do eat in a week. Apart from any you may take from the sugar bowl, note how many times you eat foods containing sugar. Not just biscuits and cakes, which are easy to avoid, but cereals, soft drinks, pickles and sauces, throat lozenges and cough linctus. Also make a note of any craving you have for it and what is happening at the time. Then it will be easier to avoid such situations in the future.

Refined sugar is also linked with bad teeth, diabetes, indigestion and thrush, and can bring on hot flushes. Is there any hope for someone with a lifelong addiction to sugar? Yes! Try cutting down gradually to wean yourself off sugar in drinks and on cereals. Try not to be tempted to use artificial sweeteners. They have their downside too. Artificial sweeteners are loaded with chemicals, such as aspartame, sodium bicarbonate, trisodium citrate, saccharin, sodium carbonate and glycine, some of which can be harmful in large doses. For example, saccharin is known to be carcinogenic and when aspartame is digested, it breaks down into methanol, which is better known as wood alcohol. When aspartame is further digested by our enzymes, it may eventually end up in our bloodstream as formaldehyde, a chemical which is used to preserve dead bodies! It has been reliably estimated that we would have to consume vast quantities of these chemical sweeteners (for example drink six hundred cans of soft drink containing aspartame within a short time) before the body is adversely affected. Nevertheless, many doctors believe that adding a daily dose of chemicals to our diet is potentially dangerous. Although the sugar in honey and carob is still sugar, these do provide other nutrients in the form of some minerals and vitamins and so can be used in moderation. Blackstrap molasses falls into this category and is a reasonable source of nutrients, but don't confuse it with golden syrup!

It is never too late to start to re-educate the taste-buds, but the longer the addiction, the longer the cure. Take it slowly and don't get discouraged. It may take some time.

SALT

Like sugar in jams, preserves and pickles, salt also entered our diet as a preservative. The châtelaine of a Norman castle and the eighteenth-century ship's purser had to supply their communities with sides of salted beef and pork to last over the winter or throughout a long voyage. Until quite recently, traditional country cookbooks would contain instructions for putting up earthenware jars of prepared runner beans between layers of salt.

Salt's scientific name is sodium chloride and it is the sodium we have to watch out for. Unlike sugar, we do need a little sodium for good nutrition. Without it there can be problems with blood, fluid balance and the nervous system. Just as a little sodium is needed for correct water balance, too much can cause water retention – a common problem. Excess sodium can block the absorption of calcium because of its similar chemical structure. But the little we need is very little, between one and three grams daily. This is what we get if we eat a good, balanced diet without the addition of any salt, either in cooking or on the table.

Besides cutting out this obvious additional salt we need to look very carefully at the content of salt in prepared food. Some things are obviously salty – crisps, peanuts and bacon – but there can also be a lot of hidden salt in quite unexpected places, such as breakfast cereals. As with sugar, the substitutes have their own disadvantages and should be treated with caution. Much better to do without. Excess salt overloads the kidneys and impairs their ability to filter fluids which can lead to water retention. Anyone suffering from bags under the eyes or swollen legs and ankles will do well to cut out added salt. Salt also raises blood pressure, hardens the arteries and upsets our hormonal balance (on top of the hormonal changes brought about by the menopause). Again, as with sugar, if you have used it for years, try cutting down what you use, first of all on the food on your plate, then in cooking and finally by avoiding salty foods. Unlike sugar, even the most addicted person is likely to find that, quite soon, foods previously enjoyed will be found too salty.

SMOKING

Now that so many facts connecting smoking with all manner of ills are apparent, no one should ever start. But the young are programmed not to listen, so there is a constant supply of smokers trying hard to give up. There are many approaches to giving up smoking and many a book written on the subject. Contact the QUIT helpline (see Useful Addresses), join an anti-smoking group, enlist the aid of your doctor, bribe yourself with the promise of a weekend at the Ritz with the money saved, anything you like – if you are a smoker, **GIVE IT UP ... NOW!**

Unfortunately, that is not the end of the list of our nutritional enemies. Here are some more.

CAFFEINE

Caffeine would quite likely be a 'banned substance' if it had been a recent discovery. It is hard to accept that the cosy mug of coffee at the kitchen table, the elegant espresso after a candlelit dinner, the frothy cappuccino at the local bistro all contain an addictive drug. Like most drugs it has its handy side, mainly one of warding off fatigue. It is much better to avoid the fatigue, or give in to it, because the downside of caffeine is greater. The price to be paid for a little increased alertness is tremendous upset in almost all areas of the body: digestion, water balance, circulation, heart rate, the pressure inside the eye. It has also been linked with an increase in fibrocystic breast pain.

If you are a great coffee drinker why not try an alternative? If you have been drinking several cups a day, and many of us have half-pint sized mugs instead of cups, wean yourself slowly, as coming off any drug can have unpleasant side-effects. These can be surprisingly strong in the case of caffeine and may cause temporary headaches.

Decaffeinated coffee, even the ground type, is readily available now and the substitutes on sale in health-food shops are good. Many people are now also turning to the great variety of herb and fruit teas which are becoming more and more popular. Start with a familiar flavour such as peppermint or blackcurrant when you need a hot drink and progress to the more exotic. Coffee is not the only source of caffeine. It is also found in considerable quantities in tea, chocolate and cola drinks, although decaffeinated forms of these can all be found.

ALCOHOL

Alcohol is another socially acceptable mind-altering drug. It, too, affects the whole physique. It obstructs the absorption of nutrients, upsets the digestive system, damages the liver and is associated with heart disease, diabetes and cancer. Despite the recent studies which indicate that small amounts of red wine are beneficial, as it contains antioxidants, alcohol is best treated with great caution.

Perhaps this section so far has cast a cloud of gloom over your view of the future, but take heart! There are very few people for whom the occasional lapse is taboo for health reasons. The vast majority of us can afford to accept the boiled sweet proffered by a small child and eat and enjoy the cholesterol-laden meal lovingly prepared by a generous hostess who has not read this *Quick Guide*. However, you owe it to yourself, and to the healthy years you have yet to enjoy, to be honest with yourself and make sure that these occasions are very much the exception.

Vitamins and Minerals

'Normal people do not need to take dietary supplements.' The discussion begins when we try to sort out what is normal. Normal people were not designed to live in an atmosphere of polluted air, travel in overcrowded, under-ventilated containers, work in stressful surroundings such long hours that they have to rely on convenient, over-refined foods. We should all, according to our physical nature, be living in spacious green countryside, growing our own fruit and vegetables, raising free-range chickens and being nice to each other. Some hope, after thousands of years of the human race trying to get away from this scenario in the cause of civilisation!

Most people describe themselves as 'about average, really'. But what is average? What we need to find out is how we each differ from the average and whether this needs attention. Enquire a little further and you will find that most average people will add something like 'but I do seem to get more than my fair share of colds' or 'if only I wasn't so tired all the time'. There is an argument as to which symptoms are a result of the menopause and which are not. Many of the 'fringe effects', while brought on by the lessening of oestrogen in the system, have no direct association with the end of fertility. However, many of these are bothersome to women going through the menopause and so have their place here.

One glance at the shelves of the health-food shop and even those of many a conventional chemist shows the extensive range of vitamins, mineral supplements and health-giving herbs now available. It's tempting to buy them all, hoping that taking one of everything will do us some good and trusting that it will do us no harm. Unfortunately it is more complicated than that.

It is well known, for example, that the mineral calcium is essential to the formation of bones and needs to be in constant supply. It has also been observed that calcium is less easily absorbed as age increases. However, too much calcium may contribute to the formation of kidney stones. From this example we can see that balanced nutrition can be a very complex business.

Vitamin D is necessary for calcium to be absorbed into the body. This is not plentiful in food. The body's main source has traditionally been sunlight, which enables the skin to manufacture it. Here is a problem also. The length of time which it is advisable to spend in the sun is particularly hard to judge, because of the risk of skin cancer. Perhaps we should take a supplement instead.

Many of the nutrients we need, and which many of us lack, are removed in the processing of food. The polishing of rice and the refining of wholemeal flour into white removes the major part of the nutritional value. We were created to eat food 'Wi' nowt taken out' in order to receive complete nutrition, but this is very difficult to achieve.

We each need to try to sort out exactly what, if any, our individual problems are. Are there headaches, joint pains, lethargy? Think what your weak points are and try to correct these, working through them one by one. Bear in mind that improvement is going to take several months in most cases. Many problems, both physical and mental, can be caused by a nutritional deficiency. It may be surprising that the taking of a simple substance in minute quantities can lift depression or anxiety. Among other symptoms which may be helped by the addition of vitamins and mineral supplements are sleeplessness, depression, poor memory and concentration, anxiety and tenseness. Add to these the physical ills which can be caused by a straightforward lack of one tiny trace of something and it can be seen that this is a huge and, as yet, imperfectly understood field of medicine.

To show how important vitamins and minerals are to us here is a brief outline of the symptoms caused by deficiencies.

Vitamins	
A and its precursor beta-carotene	Poor skin and eyesight, dry eyes and headaches.
B1	Tiredness, nausea, loss of appetite, irritability and depression.
B2	Cracked and sore lips, inflamed tongue, bloodshot or sore eyes, scaling skin, insomnia and dizziness.
B3	Muscle weakness, loss of appetite and digestive disorders, insomnia, nervousness, irritability, confusion and depression.
B5	Prematurely greying hair and hair loss.
B6	Dermatitis-like skin conditions, loss of appetite and leg cramps.
B9	Low energy levels and fatigue, irritability and confusion.
B12	Pale, grey or yellow complexion, hair loss, poor concentration and forgetfulness.
Biotin	Dermatitis and a scaling scalp.
Choline	Increase in blood fats and nerve damage.
C	Bleeding gums and poor hair growth, poor wound healing and reduced antioxidant protection.
D	Rickets in children and bone deformities. Bone softening and osteoporosis.
E	Reduced antioxidant protection and unhealthy skin.
K	Poor blood clotting.
Co-enzyme Q19	Heart malfunction.

MINERALS	
Calcium	Osteoporosis, blood clotting, muscle tone, fatigue, sleeplessness and tension.
Chromium	Blood sugar irregularities, confusion, irritability, depression, learning difficulties and thirst.
Copper	Pale skin with prominent veins, diarrhoea.
Iodine	Underactive thyroid.
Iron	Anaemia, lethargy, poor vision, indigestion, tingling fingers and toes.
Potassium	Nervousness, irritability and disorientation.
Selenium	Chest pains, hair loss and low resistance to disease.
Zinc	Low sperm count, loss of the sense of smell and taste.
AMINO ACIDS	
Cysteine	Poor absorption of selenium.
Leucine	Poor healing of skin and bones.
Lysine	Lessening of collagen.
Methionine	Poor collagen.
Valine	Neurological disorders.

These are just some of the nutrients we all need, sometimes in the minutest quantities. From the list of their effects it can be seen that many of them are particularly necessary to the middle-aged woman. For further reading, my *Quick Guide to Vitamins and Minerals* would be a good starting point. You may also like to visit a reputable nutritionist (a list can be obtained from the Society for the Promotion of Nutritional Therapy – see Useful Addresses).

6

Getting More Out of Life

Having faced up to all the difficulties that may or may not beset us during the climacteric and seeing how they can be dealt with, let us now look at the years to come. Whether you are in the throes of dealing with menopausal symptoms, past them or wondering if they are coming your way, now is a good time to think about the next stage in life.

This is a time for taking stock in all departments. There is the possibility of a change on the work front – to start, stop or change. Are there things you have always wanted to do and is this the time to say 'now or never'? Are you happy with your looks or are there improvements to be made? How is your health and fitness? Is it up to scratch to take you through your second half-century?

Many women have been described, and have even pictured themselves, only in relation to other people. This is getting rarer as more and more young women continue to work outside the home, even after the arrival of their children, but it is still frequently heard. Perhaps women now would not feel the compulsion to go on working after motherhood if they had not heard their mothers endlessly repeating 'Oh! I'm only a house-wife.' Now is the time to say 'I am myself, an independent individual', however attached you are to family and friends.

Women on their own, whether through widowhood, divorce or remaining single, often say they are made to feel pushed to the perimeter of society. Unthinking hosts often invite solitary females only to the kind of party where 'the odd woman' passes unnoticed. There are still married women to be found who consider that every single woman is a possible rival for her husband's attention. This is a highly unfair situation as a single man is considered an asset to any social occasion, even the ones who really are 'odd' men. Until we can educate society differently it is something we must find another answer for. It is especially important for women on their own to have a strong sense of their own worth.

New Interests

Work outside the home can be a major factor in helping to develop that sense of identity. It mainly falls into two categories at mid-life. Many of those who have not done it for twenty-five years want to get back into it and many who have done it all their lives are trying to work out how soon they can afford to retire. Most of us fall into one or the other category.

To get back into the world of work can take quite a bit of doing. Although ageism is not politically correct, it is rife. If you are determined to try, here are a few possibilities.

Starting to work as a volunteer in a field which interests you could lead to greater things. If earning money is not the issue, that could be enough. If you have a mature attitude to the job, turning up regularly and being dependable, you may well find that when a paid post becomes available you will be the one to get it. Similarly, if a post comes up elsewhere, you will have had recent experience and a good track record to offer which will stand you in good stead on your CV.

Starting your own business may be more than you want to contemplate but there are plenty of younger people who are doing just that and would welcome some help. Hairdressers wanting to work from home and florists setting up on their own, for example, would be grateful for a little help. Schools sometimes ask for classroom assistants to help hear the children read, take the really small to the loo and to wash grazed knees. This, too, may have to be voluntary at first but could well develop into paid work. You do not have to be an expert in the field of the person you are helping. Every employer will tell you that having an assistant who can answer the phone efficiently is an asset, and someone who can be relied upon to do whatever is needed whenever it is needed is like gold dust.

One nationwide DIY store recently had a recruiting drive to staff their stores with a large proportion of over-fifties. They have found that the older people are trustworthy, reliable and more helpful to their customers than school-leavers. Also most of them can spell and add up without a calculator. So do not believe you have nothing to offer the world of work. You may have to go out and prove it but the opportunities are there.

If you fall into the other category of looking forward to early retirement, do your sums very carefully. Retirement could be fraught if you suddenly have to watch every penny after having drawn a full-time salary for decades, but we all know of people who have worked up to their last gasp and have been too worn out to take advantage of all that terrific free time. There may be a possibility of going part time, or taking redundancy but still being on the books as a consultant – going back when work is particularly busy at audit time, the sales, or covering for holiday time or maternity leave.

If there is anything you have always wished you could do, now is the time to try. From learning to do patchwork to pot-holing to playing the piano, have a go. Dr Margaret Rule, who did so much in the raising of Henry VIII's warship, the *Mary Rose*, learnt deep-sea diving in her forties. Women have taken up long-distance running, golf, gone on playing high-level tennis well into their later years. The secret is to take things to your own level. Do not forgo the pleasure of learning to play a musical instrument just because you will never get into a symphony orchestra.

Singing can be taken up at any age and there are choirs everywhere for all standards and tastes. Dancing, too, gives a lot of pleasure and together with singing is good news physically. Do not be afraid to take up something which needs concentration. If you feel you have enough to think about with your day-to-day worries, this is just the time to embark upon something which will take you right out of yourself. An hour and a half trying to fit the words, or the feet, to the music in the company of others and having a good laugh when it all goes awry is refreshing beyond belief.

If your memory has become poor a good way of helping it is to take up a course of study. This may sound contradictory, but memory is improved with regular use. Learning a language, especially in the company of others, can be fun as well as 'improving'. It can also lead to other interests, such as international affairs, travel, pen-friendships.

Anything which broadens our horizons is a good thing. The Open University is often in the news. It is not necessary to plunge straight into a degree course. They have plenty of short courses of great variety which really can be studied wherever you are and whatever your situation. Many local colleges of further education have Access courses, helping people back into studying and have open evenings which anyone can attend with no obligation.

On a more everyday scale, to help your memory try remembering the items you have to get at the supermarket. Then, when you check with your list you will be able to note your improvement. Try remembering the addresses of friends when you write your Christmas cards and only look in your address book later. Memory can improve with use, but like any exercise, it has to be worked at.

A Physical Rethink

Nobody needs to be told that their looks change as time goes by. Only if you believe that to be beautiful you have to be young is this a cause for sadness. Do not give in to this brainwashing, stand up and fight!

CLOTHES

Nothing is more ageing than a middle-aged woman wearing the styles that she wore at seventeen. These are thirty years out of date and she runs the risk of becoming 'mutton dressed as lamb'. We have to come to terms with the fact that we can no longer throw on jeans and a T-shirt, tie our greying locks into a pony-tail and look a million dollars. This is not to say that you must throw out all your old favourites, however idiosyncratic, just that they may be improved by a little updating. If you are not interested in looking a million dollars, fine; but if you are and are not sure how to achieve it, now might be the time to visit a style and colour consultant. Some are more expensive than others, most will come to your home and some will organise evenings for three or four friends. There are also books on the subject, one of the most comprehensive being Mary Spillane's *Complete Style Guide*.

How you look is important to achieving what you want out of life. If we want to get across the message 'I am a mature person, wise in the ways of the world and have a lot to offer society' we have to look the part. Politicians are told that they have thirty seconds in which to make their desired impression on TV viewers. It is estimated that what people think of us at first meeting is based 5 percent on what we say, 10 percent on how we say it and 85 percent on how we look. So first impressions are vital if we are to go back to work or take up a more public life than before. Besides, it is fun to have a change.

We have all got so used to picking up our usual sized bra from the chainstore shelf it may have slipped our notice that it no longer fits as well as it used to. A visit to a specialist shop with a qualified fitter could be very profitable. However, don't be tempted to buy over-supportive corsets. It is much better to work at toning up your muscles.

HAIR

Hair style makes a great impact. How often have you not at first recognised a familiar face because the haircut has changed? Beside employing the 'be kind to your tresses' methods described in Chapter 2, do not be afraid to experiment with different styles. Even if you make a mistake, the consoling thing about hair is that even the worst of horrors will grow out.

HANDS AND FEET

Nails can become brittle with lack of oestrogen and while they are in this state it is better to avoid using nail varnish. The varnish itself is not so damaging, but the remover can be drying. Try grooming your nails with cream polishes and a chamois leather buffer after filing. Keeping the circulation good can go a long way to preventing the nails, both on fingers and toes, from thickening to the point that they become difficult to cut. Think of adding a regular visit to the chiropodist to your list of health checks.

The state of our feet is reflected in our faces so it is important to keep them happy if we are to present a smiling face to the world. Four-inch stilettos have never been a good idea for feet, legs or wooden floors. There is no doubt that a higher heel flatters the ankle but they don't have to be that high to achieve this effect, and a wide base to the heel helps balance. It may sound odd, but it is a good idea to buy shoes at the end of a day's shopping when you are hot and tired and your feet are swollen. If the new shoes are comfortable then, they always will be.

Indoors, go without shoes as much as possible. Sit with your feet raised to drain fluid from your ankles. Take special care of any cuts or sore places on the feet and legs. If blood circulation is poor, lower limbs are slower to heal. Tight footwear, shoes or stockings, can cause poor circulation, cold feet and chilblains. Avoid long soaking in hot water because it will soften the skin and leave a moist surface for infections to develop. Have the bath just comfortably warm. After drying well, massage the feet with hand lotion.

TEETH

Your teeth are likely to be less trouble now than they were in our earlier years. Mouth problems are more likely to be centred around the gums. Lack of collagen can cause receding gums, and the long-toothed look of many older people. Regular, frequent brushing is very important to remove plaque which is associated with the common gum disease, pyorrhoea, and the consequent loss of good teeth. Cosmetic dental work is very effective in maintaining the shape of the face, but it is far better to avoid the need for it by ever more rigorous daily dental hygiene.

EYES

Some people are reluctant to take to wearing glasses for reading because they feel it is ageing. Unfortunately there is no disguising the fact that they cannot read the telephone directory because their arms are not long enough to hold it sufficiently far away. Bifocal glasses are a real give-away but it is now possible to get lenses that graduate from long-distance correction at the top to reading strength at the bottom without a noticeable horizontal line. The top part can be plain glass so that those who do not need correction of their long-distance vision can have glasses that they can wear all day, which saves a lot of hunting around. Bifocal contact lenses are also available.

Annual eye tests are important even if there seems to be no deterioration in sight. Opticians can detect early signs of diseases such as high blood pressure and glaucoma before they make themselves felt. Dry eye is a condition which is very uncomfortable but common in the post-menopausal. It can be improved by the prescription of 'artificial tears', and bathing the eyes with a mild infusion of the herb eyebright can be soothing.

BREASTS

Every woman, old or young, on HRT or not, should check her breasts regularly, making a habit of doing it on the first of every month if you have stopped menstruating. If you have not stopped, the end of your period is the best time. That is when your breasts are likely to be at their least lumpy for reasons of hormonal change. All doctors' surgeries and health centres these days have detailed leaflets on how to do a thorough examination. Basically it is best to lie down on your back with one hand behind your head. With the other hand systematically feel the opposite breast, pressing gently but firmly in a circular motion. Feel also for any lumps in the armpit and along the collar bone. Repeat on the opposite side. Standing in front of a mirror look out for any signs of dimpling, puckering or an inverted nipple. If in any doubt about any of your findings go to the doctor without delay for the 90 percent certain reassurance it is likely to be, or the early action needed if the situation warrants it. Any discharge from the nipple also needs medical attention.

Mammography is becoming more common, and every time one is offered it should probably be taken up. A mammogram will reveal the minute beginnings of tumours if any are present while they are still far too small to be detected manually. Cervical smear tests are also still important to keep up to date, even though the likelihood of cervical cancer diminishes as the years go by.

If you have back or joint pain your doctor may recommend that you have a bone density scan. This, like mammography, is a type of X-ray. It is a technique for the early discovery of osteoporosis and checking on its development. Some studies associate early greying of hair with the onset of osteoporosis, so this may be an additional warning sign.

Exercise

Nutrition plays an enormously important part in health and fitness, both mental and physical, as we have seen in the previous chapter, but another contributory factor is exercise. There are exercises for easing almost every symptom we might suffer from as a result of passing through the menopause.

Good posture is essential to give an appearance of the vigorous good health we all want. It helps to keep the spine in shape which in turn means that the rest of the body is in the best position. Lie down on the floor and see if you can ease every bone of your spine down to touch the floor. If the middle of your back arches up at the waist, bend your knees. Lower the legs until the vertebrae start to rise. With practice you will be nearer and nearer to being able to lie absolutely flat, as the back muscles get stronger and the joints more flexible.

One way to check that your posture is correct is to imagine that you have a hook right on the top of your head. Imagine that someone is holding you up by it like a marionette. That way, your neck will lengthen, your shoulders will drop down and back and you will walk like a ballerina. Only, unlike a ballerina keep your feet pointing directly forward, as turning the feet out will make you waddle.

If you are really stiff, a good way back to flexibility is to spend a few weeks going to the toning tables. These move the different areas of the body as gently and slowly as you wish. You can work with the movements or, as you get stronger, resist them. They will not lose weight for you, and they will not make you fit but they will strengthen your muscles and loosen your joints. It can be expensive, but in two or three months, you will be in a much better state to take on a more vigorous and less pricey regime of exercise.

Exercise to keep the weight down depends on burning up calories and really has to be combined with a sensible diet. Keeping the heart in trim depends on making the heart work a little overtime. We can tell when this is happening because the blood in our veins begins to flow and we get pink cheeks, warm fingers and toes and a little out of breath. However, it is important not to take exercise to the point where you feel pain or are too out of breath to speak. Take it easy – you will soon build up the amount you can do.

Any exercise which really gets you going will do, the choice is yours: from a brisk walk for thirty minutes or so three times a week, to a keep-fit class, to going to a gym and engaging the services of a personal trainer, all these are good. Low-impact aerobics is better than a lot of leaping around which could very well be too much for middle-aged joints, especially if they are carrying too much weight. The same goes for jogging to begin with. Dancing can be fun and sociable too.

It has been discovered that exercising to a point where your pulse is only moderately raised is more efficient at burning fat than when you are puffing and blowing. This is because at the higher level you are taking in less oxygen, and it is the oxygen that burns up fat. Exercising at a moderate level means that the weight you lose will be made up of fat and will not be lost muscle.

To increase the fitness of the heart and circulation you need to exercise more briskly. All muscles strengthen after being made to work hard regularly, and this is also true of the muscles of the heart. It is still important not to overdo the exercising to the point of pain and exhaustion. As you lose the weight and gain strength and fitness you will be able to branch out into other fields. To start with, limit yourself to getting really warm and slightly puffed at each session. When exercising keep your tummy tucked in. Not only does it look better, it stops your internal organs from bouncing about and possibly being damaged.

The exercises for weight control and the heart are also good for the prevention of osteoporosis at least in the lower limbs. Different forms of exercise have to be added to give strength to the upper spine and shoulders. Swimming is often held as the perfect exercise and so it is from the point of view of flexibility, but not for osteoporosis. The same is true of cycling. What improves the consistency of bone is weight-bearing exercise. Games like tennis and badminton are excellent, as would be a programme of gentle weight training (not to be confused with weight lifting!). If you belong to a gym, or go to classes, ask the instructor to show you how to use weights or dumb bells. You can buy weighted wrist-bands for use at home or even make the movements holding tins of beans! You do need to be shown how to do the exercises safely, however, to avoid injury. Linda Ojeda's *Menopause without Medicine* has a very good section on exercise.

Even if osteoporosis has already set in, the condition will improve with exercise and good diet, even, to a certain extent, without HRT. However, a sufferer should take especial care not to strain, especially when making movements that involve the spine. Forget 'pushing through the pain barrier', though. That may be right for candidates for the next Olympic hurdling team but it is not for us normal mortals. Stress is what activates the osteoblast cells into building new bone, but it can be overdone.

Bones and muscles both improve with use. Exercise not only strengthens us, it improves co-ordination and lessens the likelihood of us breaking bones in a fall caused by overbalancing. Exercising while losing weight helps to reduce the slackness of the skin as the fat disappears from under it. The increase in circulation also improves its colour and texture.

Exercises for helping with incontinence could not be simpler. When you next spend a penny, stop in mid flow, start again and stop once more. Contract these muscles at any time of the day. Do it as often as you remember. This will increase your control greatly.

Sagging breasts can be lifted by an increase in the muscle tone attained by the exercises for the upper body generally. Another exercise, which can be done at any time, is clasping the hands together at chin level and, raising the elbows so that the arms are parallel with the ground, pushing the hands together in a series of pulses. You will see the effect as the muscles supporting the bust are flexed.

Rest

Many older people claim to be plagued by insomnia. Unless you wake up exhausted, this may not actually be the case. We need less sleep as we age, although the reasons for this are not altogether known. If you find you cannot get to sleep at what you have always thought of as your usual time, wake up early or have an hour or two of wakefulness in the middle of the night, this may be the explanation. Regard it as bonus time. How often have we complained there are not enough hours in the day? Even the middle of the night can be useful for planning, as long as it is not of a worrying type. The quality of sleep is more important than the quantity. In fact quite a lot of useful rest can be gained while awake, in the middle of the night or at any other time. Exercising will also help insomnia – studies have shown that the fit have better sleep patterns than the unfit.

To stop the mind racing and as part of relaxation, keep the jaw and tongue loose. It is remarkable how this will stop the flow of 'what I should have said, done, remembered' which plagues us all, especially in the dark hours.

If this all sounds as if exercise is the cure to all our ills it is because the vast majority of people in the modern world do not get nearly the amount we are built to take.

Stress in the right amount is good for us all. It makes life exciting, keeps us on our toes and gives us interesting problems to solve. An overdose of stress is not so good. Relaxation techniques help as do yoga, meditation and prayer. Stressful situations which arise suddenly, shocks or frights are helped by a few drops of Bach's Rescue Remedy on the tongue. The Bach flower remedies were discovered and developed in the last century and the Rescue Remedy is probably the most widely known and used. They can be found in health-food shops and in some chemists and come in tiny brown dropper bottles, handy for carrying around.

Illness and injury can be stressful and rest is very important in getting over them. When doctors prescribe 'bed rest', it is not because they can't think of anything else! Like all living things we are programmed to heal, to be whole. Blood starts to clot in a cut finger at once. It does not wait until you have run it under the tap and found the sticking plaster. A broken bone begins to heal instantly, not after the orthopaedic surgeon has examined the X-rays. Healing is a wonderful process but it takes energy. The best way to help it is to go easy on yourself. Forget 'bravely soldiering on' when you have the 'flu. You will get better quicker and more completely if you rest.

So, there is much to be decided and done. The menopausal years, the climacteric, are a busy time of reassessment and adjustment. If all this sounds as if it is going to take some time and effort, well, perhaps it is, but this is as it should be. To have a happy, healthy remainder of your life needs care but it will pay off. If you feel guilty about spending time on yourself remember that the healthier you are, the less trouble you will be to others and everyone will benefit.

Glossary

Acupuncture – a traditional Chinese system of healing that involves the use of thin metal needles which are inserted into specific points beneath the skin to relieve symptoms.

Aromatherapy – the therapeutic use of herbal essential oils to treat many kinds of disorders, notably hormonal problems, skin complaints and stress.

Climacteric – the medical name for the three stages of the menopause, essentially meaning when a woman has her last period.

Cranial osteopathy – helps to heal disorders by realigning the bones in the skull.

Endometriosis – the state when tissue, similar to the lining of the womb, forms inside the uterus and other areas of the pelvis.

Fibroids – a benign tumour or growth of fibrous tissue which may develop in the wall of the uterus.

Herbalism – a natural form of medicine which uses various parts of plants to relieve certain conditions.

HRT – Hormone Replacement Therapy.

Incontinence – the involuntary release of urine from the bladder.

Oestrogen – one of the female hormones, also used in HRT.

Osteoporosis – a degenerative disease caused by thinning of the bones and a loss of bone mass over time.

Progesterone – another of the female hormones, also used in HRT.

Reflexology – a form of therapeutic foot massage where each part of the foot corresponds to a different part of the body.

Shiatsu – a form of therapeutic massage involving a rhythmic series of finger pressures over the entire body.

Yoga – an ancient spiritual practice from India that aims to tone the mind, body and soul through various moving and static poses and exercises, breathing exercises, diet and meditation.

Useful Addresses

Breast Cancer Care
15–19 Britten Street
London SW3 3TZ
Helpline: 0171-867 1103
Specialises in all aspects of breast cancer.

British Heart Foundation
14 Fitzhardinge Street
London W1H 4DH
Tel: 0171-935 0185
Send an SAE for information on prevention of heart disease and all aspects of heart problems.

British Homoeopathic Association
27a Devonshire Street
London W1N 1RJ
Tel: 0171-935 2163
They have nationwide lists of conventionally trained doctors who have completed postgraduate training in homoeopathy.

British School of Reflexology
92 Sheering Road
Old Harlow CM17 0JW
Tel: 01279 429060
Send an SAE for a list of qualified practitioners.

British Wheel of Yoga
1 Hamilton Place
Boston Road
Sleaford NG34 7ES
Tel: 01529 306851
Send an SAE for a nationwide list of qualified teachers.

Carers' National Association
20/25 Glasshouse Yard
London EC1A 4JS
Helpline: 0171-490 8818
They will put carers in touch with local support groups and can give advice on how to get respite care, what financial benefits are available, how to apply for it and all other aspects of caring for the elderly or disabled in the home.

Continence Foundation
c/o The Dene Centre
Castle Farm Road
Newcastle upon Tyne NE3 1PH
Helpline: 0191-213 0050
Offer advice on all types of incontinence, bladder and bowel. Send an SAE for information.

Council for Acupuncture
179 Gloucester Place
London NW1 6DX
Tel: 0171-724 5756
Contact for details of qualified practitioners near you or send £2.50 for a nationwide directory.

General Council and Register of Osteopaths Ltd
56 London Street
Reading RG1 4SQ
Tel: 01734 576585

Endometriosis Society
35 Belgrave Square
London SW1X 8QB
Tel: 0171-235 4137

International Federation of Aromatherapists
Stamford House
2/4 Chiswick High Road
London W4 1TH
Tel: 0181 742 2605
Send an SAE for a list of qualified practitioners near you.

Margaret Pyke Centre
15 Bateman's Buildings
Soho Square
London W1V 6JB
Tel: 0171-734 9351
Offer complete assessment for suitability for HRT and the necessary medication. No need for referral by a GP and no charge except for prescriptions, although donations are welcomed as this organisation relies on voluntary contributions.

Marie Stopes Centre
108 Whitfield Street
London W1P 6BE
Tel: 0171-388 2585
(and also in Leeds and Manchester)
Offer a fifty-minute 'Menocheck' to assess hormone levels, general health and suitability for HRT. There is no need for referral by a GP but there is a charge of £100 for the check-up and for any prescriptions.

National Institute of Herbalists
56 Longbrook Street
Exeter EX4 6AH
Tel: 01392 426022
They have lists of qualified herbalists nationwide.

National Osteoporosis Society
PO Box 10
Radstock
Bath BA3 3YB
Tel: 01761 432472
Send an SAE for information.

Open University
Central Enquiry Service
PO Box 200
Milton Keynes MK7 6YZ
Tel: 01908 653231

QUIT
Victory House
170 Tottenham Court Road
London W1P 0HA
Tel: 0171-487 3000
A helpline to give support to those wishing to break the smoking habit.

Research into Ovarian Cancer (ROC)
PO Box 387
London SW15 1XR
Tel: 0181-789 1406

Samaritans
Tel: 0171-734 2800 (in London; local numbers in all telephone directories)
Befriend the suicidal.

Shiatsu Society
5 Foxcote
Wokingham
Berkshire RG11 3PL
Tel: 01734 730836 (Mondays, Tuesdays and Fridays 2–5pm, or leave a message on their answering machine)
Provide a list of qualified practitioners in your area.

Society for the Promotion of Nutritional Therapy (SPNT)
1st Floor, The Enterprise Centre
Station Parade
Eastbourne BN21 1BE
Tel: 01323 430203
Send an SAE for information.

Society of Homoeopaths
2 Artisan Road
Northampton NN1 4HU
Tel: 01604 21400
They have nationwide lists of qualified lay homoeopaths.

Weight Watchers UK Ltd
Kidwells PK House
Kidwells PK Drive
Maidenhead
London W1X 8HB
Tel: 0171-491 1929

Women's Health

Helpline: 0171-251 6580 (between 10am and 4pm on
Mondays, Wednesdays, Thursdays and Fridays)
53 Featherstone Street
London EC1Y 8RT

*They deal with all women's health problems, not just cancer. Their
resource centre, which is open for the same hours as the helpline,
can be visited without appointment and has books and information
covering all aspects of women's health. They are also able to put
people in touch with support groups for all manner of problems.*

Women's Nationwide Cancer Control Campaign

Helpline: 0171-729 2229

*They will answer any questions on cancer, its diagnosis,
treatment and aftercare, etc.*

Further Reading

Liz Earle's *Quick Guides* to *Evening Primrose Oil, Food Combining, Successful Slimming* and *Vitamins and Minerals*, all published by Boxtree (£3.99 each).

The Complete Style Guide, Mary Spillane (Piatkus, £14.95).

Hormone Replacement Therapy, Rosemary Nicol (Vermilion, £6.99).

HRT and the Menopause, Dr R C D Wilson (Consumers' Association and Hodder & Stoughton, £9.99).

Menopause, Dr Miriam Stoppard (Dorling Kindersley, £14.99).

Menopause, The Best Years of Your Life, Ada Kahn and Linda Hughey Holt (Bloomsbury, £4.99).

Menopause without Medicine, Linda Ojeda (Thorsons, £4.99).

The Silent Passage, Gail Sheehy (HarperCollins, £5.99).

The Tofu Cookbook, Leah Leneman (Thorsons, £5.99).

Index

HOW TO ORDER YOUR BOXTREE BOOKS BY LIZ EARLE

Liz Earl's Quick Guides

Available Now

❑ 1 85283 542 7	Aromatherapy	£3.99
❑ 1 85283 544 3	Baby and Toddler Foods	£3.99
❑ 1 85283 543 5	Food Facts	£3.99
❑ 1 85283 546 X	Vegetarian Cookery	£3.99
❑ 0 7522 1619 8	Evening Primrose Oil	£3.99
❑ 0 7533 1614 7	Herbs for Health	£3.99
❑ 1 85283 984 8	Successful Slimming	£3.99
❑ 1 85283 989 9	Vitamins and Minerals	£3.99
❑ 1 85283 979 1	Detox	£3.99
❑ 0 7522 1635 X	Hair Loss	£3.99
❑ 0 7522 1636 8	Youthful Skin	£3.99
❑ 0 7522 1680 5	Healthy Pregnancy	£3.99
❑ 0 7522 1636 8	Dry Skin and Eczema	£3.99
❑ 0 7522 1641 4	Cod Liver Oil	£3.99
❑ 0 7522 1626 0	Juicing	£3.99

Coming Soon

❑ 0 7522 1645 7	Beating Cellulite	£3.99
❑ 0 7522 1673 2	Food Combining	£3.99
❑ 0 7522 1690 2	Post-natal Health	£3.99
❑ 0 7522 1675 9	Food Allergies	£3.99
❑ 0 7522 1685 6	Healthy Menopause	£3.99
❑ 0 7522 1668 6	Beating PMS	£3.99
❑ 0 7522 1663 5	Antioxidants	£3.99

ACE Plan Titles

❑ 1 85283 518 4	Liz Earle's Ace Plan The New Guide to Super Vitamins A, C and E	£4.99
❑ 1 85283 554 0	Liz Earle's Ace Plan Weight-Loss for Life	£4.99

All the books shown on the previous page are available at your local bookshop or can be ordered direct from the publisher. Just tick the titles you want and fill in the form below. Prices and availability subject to change without notice.

Boxtree Cash Sales,
PO Box 11, Falmouth, Cornwall TR10 9EN

Please send cheque or postal order for the value of the book(s), and add the following for postage and packing:

UK including BFPO – £1.00 for one book, plus 50p for the second book, and 30p for each additional book ordered up to a £3.00 maximum.
Overseas including Eire – £2.00 for the first book, plus £1.00 for the second book, and 50p for each additional book ordered.

OR
please debit this amount from my Access/VISA card (delete as appropriate)

Card number ☐☐☐☐☐☐☐☐☐☐☐☐☐☐☐☐☐☐

Amount £...

Expiry date on card ....

Signed ....

Name ....

Address ....

....

....